# Sleep and Learning

## The Magic that Makes Us Healthy and Smart

Gary R. Plaford

Rowman & Littlefield Education
Lanham • New York • Toronto • Plymouth, UK

Published in the United States of America
by Rowman & Littlefield Education
A Division of Rowman & Littlefield Publishers, Inc.
A wholly owned subsidary of The Rowman & Littlefield Publishing Group, Inc.
4501 Forbes Boulevard, Suite 200, Lanham, Maryland 20706
www.rowmaneducation.com

Estover Road
Plymouth PL6 7PY
United Kingdom

British Cataloging in Publication Information Available

**Library of Congress Cataloging-in-Publication Data**

Plaford, Gary R., 1947-
  Sleep and learning : the magic that makes us healthy and smart / Gary R.
Plaford.
      p. cm.
  Includes bibliographical references and index.
  ISBN 978-1-60709-091-5 (cloth : alk. paper) — ISBN 978-1-60709-092-2 (pbk. :
alk. paper) — ISBN 978-1-60709-093-9 (electronic)
  1. Sleep. I. Title.
  QP425.P53 2009
  612.8'21—dc22                                                    2009003869

# Contents

# Preface

When I tell some of my friends and colleagues that I am working on a book on sleep I get some interesting questions. Actually I usually get the same question, but the emphasis is different. "*Why* are you writing a book on sleep?" "Why are *you* writing a book on sleep?" "Why are you writing a book on *sleep*?" The implication is that they are somehow questioning my credentials in this area.

The truth is, I have slept, and at times I have slept well. I like to remind some of my colleagues of the times they walked into my office and I might have had my feet up, my eyes might have been closed, and there was possibly the hint of a slight snore escaping my air passage. That, I state defiantly, was research. I have put in hours of research.

Seriously, regardless of the emphasis, the question is a good one. My decision to write this book did not occur suddenly. The road to this decision took several turns. Let me explain. I am recently retired from my long-standing position as director of Social Services for the Monroe County Community School Corporation. I continue to teach classes at Indiana University in Bloomington on understanding and dealing with youth and adolescents and on understanding and working with organizations. I have a book, published in 2006, entitled *Bullying and the Brain: Using Cognitive and Emotional Intelligence to Help Kids Cope.*

I also have done, and continue to do, a lot of speaking at school corporations, with school faculties, and at conferences on issues related to bullying and brain research and/or poverty and brain research. Last year

I spoke at numerous conferences including "The Learning and the Brain Conference" in Boston, Massachusetts, and at "The Oxford Round Table" held at Oxford University in Oxford, England.

These interests have caused me to do a great deal of reading about the brain and how it functions, including what happens under stress and with post-traumatic stress disorder. That was my first brush with the topic of sleep. Post-traumatic stress disorder is experienced by people who experience a traumatic event but also who have experienced disrupted REM (rapid eye movement) sleep and have therefore not processed the experience. REM sleep, or the lack of REM sleep, is a key issue in this disorder. I kept reading.

Other mental and emotional disorders that people experience including schizophrenia, bipolar disorder, and depression are related to stress but are also related to sleep issues. For a long time we have known that sleep issues are symptoms of these disorders, but it is becoming evident that sleep is much more involved than as merely a symptom. I kept reading.

Physical issues are also related to sleep. Fibromyalgia, for one, is certainly related to decreased slow wave sleep. New research is linking sleep, and the ongoing deprivation of sleep, to issues like cancer and diabetes. This is because sleep is linked to such things as the functioning of the immune system and the release of growth hormone. I kept reading.

Memory storage and recall are also linked to sleep. The first major study that really linked sleep to memory was released just fourteen years ago. Before that there were researchers studying sleep and researchers studying memory, but they were not on the same page. We now know there are critical links between the two. There are some different theories about what is actually going on because it really is a new frontier. I was fascinated, and I continued to read.

Another issue that is related is that of dreams. There are certainly some different views as to the function and purpose of dreams. I could not put the books and journals down.

At some point around this time I found that because of my previous reading about such things as brain functioning, stress, managing stress, the fight or flight response, and so forth, I had some opinions about some of the theories out there. I tended to agree with some and strongly disagree with others. I also shared some of the information I was reading with friends and colleagues in informal discussions. I found that they were enthralled with the subject of sleep and the multiple issues related to sleep, and at the same time limited in knowledge about the subject.

This is when I decided to put down the books and pick up the pen. There is much that has been learned about sleep in just the past few years, but the average citizen knows very little about the topic. I wanted to change that. This is not merely interesting information, it is critical information. Because sleep affects mental health, physical health, how we function in life, memory and learning, it has a tremendous impact on education.

The gradual and cumulative sleep deprivation that many students endure not only makes them too tired to focus well, but it also hampers memory consolidation and motivation. If we really want to improve school performance and graduation rates we cannot afford to overlook something as basic and critical as sleep. Additionally, if we want to make an impact on both the physical and mental health of individuals in our society (which impacts mortality rates, health care, health insurance rates, the aging process, etc.) we need to begin by educating our youth about the relevance of sleep on these issues.

All that I have read has changed my perspective on sleep, my perspective about the need to educate parents, educators, and students about the importance of sleep, and my own behaviors related to sleep. My hope is to share this information in a concise and readable format so that others, especially educators and parents, have the knowledge to make whatever changes they might find helpful and necessary for children. That, I suppose, answers the question, *"Why are you writing a book on sleep?"*

# Chapter 1

# Introduction

*There is a common saying, "If I hadn't seen it I wouldn't have believed it." The interesting thing is that the reverse of that saying is also true, "If I hadn't believed it I wouldn't have seen it." The fact is we organize the information in our world based on what we know or think we know. We cannot organize it any other way. When we look at something we do not all see the same thing, we do not see an objectively real world that everyone else sees, we see what is meaningful to us. Perception is always dependent on meaning, always about meaning. There are facts . . . there are truths. However, the most critical aspect of perception lies not in the facts themselves, but rather in how we interpret those facts.*

*When we see a movie, some of us may like it, some may love it, some may hate it. We perceive the movie based on our own past experiences, our own beliefs, our own interpretations. We do not, in effect, see the same movie. There is no objective reality, there are only similarities. First of all, we only perceive a small amount of the sensory information that is available to us, and secondly, all that we do perceive is based on our own individual interpretations, and that is limited by what we already know. All that we perceive in the world is ultimately based on our own, individual perspective.*

There is a vast store of knowledge that has currently and is continually being amassed on the subject of sleep. There is still a great deal to learn, but from what has already been learned we know that it is much more important than we realized. Most people believe that the function of sleep is merely to rest. Although that is one function of sleep, it is only one. There

1

is a lot more going on in our brains and in our bodies when we close our eyes at night. When we deprive ourselves of sleep, or of the proper levels of the different stages of sleep, we begin to have problems . . . sometimes significant problems.

When children and adolescents don't get the levels of sleep they need they have these same problems, as well as the added issue that it hampers their education in multiple ways. The very basic task of growing up is to learn. . .to get an education. That is what allows children to eventually take their place as a functioning member of the adult world. If that process is being hampered, we need to address the reasons why.

The purpose of this book is to explain sleep, what goes on during sleep, what happens when we have sleep deprivation or sleep problems, what we can do to improve sleep, and what we need to know and to do in order to help our children sleep better. The quantity and quality of sleep that our children and our students get significantly impacts their ability to learn and to function in their world. Sleep is much more significant than we thought.

There are a number of issues and questions that will be addressed through this book. These will include a discussion about the stages of sleep and what they entail. It will address rapid-eye-movement (REM) sleep and non-REM sleep, how we cycle through these stages during the night, and what happens when we don't get appropriate levels of these cycles. Different things happen in our brains and our bodies during the different stages of sleep. So, what are some of these crucial functions? What occurs during non-REM sleep? What occurs specifically during what is called slow wave sleep, which is collectively sleep stages three and four of non-REM?

How is the immune system affected by sleep and/or sleep deprivation? How does sleep impact our body's ability to maintain heat? How does sleep affect metabolism and body weight? What is the relationship between sleep deprivation and diabetes, or sleep deprivation and cancer? Can working the night shift year after year cause enough sleep deprivation to affect the body's ability to ward off cancer?

What is sleep apnea? What effect does sleep apnea have on blood pressure and heart disease? Can sleep apnea result in weight gain? Is it possible that some of the diagnoses of attention-deficit/hyperactivity disorder (ADHD) are really caused by sleep apnea?

What is the function of REM sleep? Why is it critical? What is the relationship of REM sleep to memory? What is memory? Is there a difference between memory storage and memory retrieval? Memory is a critical aspect of learning. Memory is what learning is all about. Is it any wonder that sleep problems or sleep deprivation will impact a child's memory and hence his education?

What is the relationship between REM sleep and depression? How many depressed adolescents are we seeing? What are the consequences when depressed individuals get more REM sleep and less slow wave sleep?

What is the relationship between REM sleep and schizophrenia? Some of the symptoms of mental psychoses are sleep difficulties, but are sleep problems more than merely symptoms of these psychoses?

What happens with our muscles during REM sleep? Have you ever awakened to find that for just a brief moment you were paralyzed? Is it possible that the muscle paralysis naturally experienced during REM sleep is also related to catatonic schizophrenia?

What is the relationship between REM sleep and post-traumatic stress disorder? Why do the traumatic emotions of post-traumatic stress disorder continually come flooding back to the individual exactly as they were experienced?

What are dreams really all about? Why do we dream? What do we dream about? What is the significance of the fact that we dream?

Why is it that sometimes when we "sleep on a problem" it resolves itself? Why do we have insights and solutions to issues after we sleep when we couldn't seem to figure it out during our waking hours?

Is there any possible relationship between sleep deprivation and abuse and neglect? How is behavior influenced by sleep?

What is the relationship between aging and sleep? Our memories don't function as well as we grow old. We tend to have more aches and pains as we grow old. We become more unsteady on our feet and fall more easily as we grow old. Are these simply related to the fact that we are older, or are they related to the fact that we are also getting less REM sleep and less sleep overall? Can we impact the aging process by how we currently address sleep?

What is the circadian clock that ticks inside each of us? How does this internal time mechanism affect sleep, and how can it be altered or impacted by sleep problems? Why are some people morning people and some night people, and why is it that adolescents tend to become night people during the teenage years?

What is the relationship of stress to sleep? What are the conditions that cause stress? What goes on in the brain when we undergo stress? What are the levels of stress and what happens when we experience fight or flight? How can we manage stress and teach our children to manage stress in order to improve sleep?

How do the left and right hemispheres of the brain work in relation to the tasks they perform? How is that important in understanding how the locus of control of brain functions can shift? How can we learn to shift the locus of control of our own brain functioning and teach our children to do so to calm themselves and embrace sleep easier?

What strategies and techniques can we incorporate to achieve more sleep overall as well as more qualitative sleep? What can be done for those individuals who wake up during the night and have trouble returning to sleep? Can napping be part of the solution and, if so, exactly how?

What is the relationship between sleep and learning, concentration, memory, focus, and behavior . . . all critical in achieving a quality education? If sleep is so important, and the proper levels of REM and non-REM sleep are so critical, what can we do to teach our children about the importance of sleep? How can we teach our children to better manage stress and achieve sleep easier for both improved mental and physical health, and to help them be more productive?

These are some of the issues and questions that will be addressed in this book. It is important to first understand the functions of sleep and how these functions, when disrupted, impact our lives. With that knowledge we can then perceive our world from a somewhat different perspective, and come to a better understanding of how we can make this world a better, healthier, saner, and more productive place for children to grow and learn.

# Chapter 2

# The Stages of Sleep— What's It All About?

*An old priest and an old bus driver, neither functioning in their jobs as well as they had when they were younger men, both ended up dying on the same day. They were greeted at the pearly gates by St. Peter. St. Peter gave the old bus driver the keys to a brand new Cadillac.*

*"Here you are," said St. Peter. "This is yours to travel around heaven for all eternity."*

*The bus driver was delighted and quickly drove away in his new car. St. Peter turned to the old priest and held up a pair of roller skates.*

*"And here you are," he said to the priest. "This will get you around heaven for all eternity."*

*The priest was dismayed.*

*"But. . .but. . .but," he said, "I was a priest. I had a congregation. Why does that bus driver get a Cadillac and I only get roller skates?"*

*"It has to do with your productivity for the Lord while on earth," said St. Peter.*

*"But I preached to my congregation every Sunday," argued the priest.*

*"When you preached to your congregation you put them to sleep. When he drove, people prayed!"*

There are many jokes about sleep, and we all have conversations about sleep. "I didn't sleep well last night," or "Boy, what a great night's sleep I got." But what is sleep really all about? What happens when we put our heads on that pillow and close our eyes? Is it merely about resting our brains and our bodies? If it were merely about rest, then why do we go through so many different levels of sleep, and why do these levels repeat as cycles all night long?

In reality there are five stages of sleep (Mednick 2006, 33–44). There are four stages of non-REM sleep, simply called stages 1, 2, 3, and 4, and one stage of REM sleep. When we first begin to sleep we enter stage 1 of non-REM sleep. This is light sleep. We may drift in and out of light sleep and we can be awakened fairly easily during this stage. Stage 1 typically lasts only one to five minutes and occurs only at the beginning of the sleep cycle. Stage 1 has been described as a quasi-REM state, but without the rapid eye movement. It acts as sort of a warm-up for sleep.

After that we move into stage 2 non-REM sleep. During this stage eye movement stops, brain waves become slower, the heart rate slows, and the body temperature drops. Brain waves, though slower, are interspersed with occasional bursts called spindles. The first time we go into stage 2 during the night it will last somewhere between ten to fifteen minutes. Subsequent stage 2 periods will last only five to seven minutes. Stage 2 is the go-between for the other stages. In other words we go from stage 2 to slow wave sleep (stages 3 and 4), then back through stage 2, then to REM, then back through stage 2, then slow wave again, then back through stage 2, then REM, and so forth throughout the night.

As we progress to stage 3 of non-REM sleep extremely slow brain waves begin to appear. These very slow waves are called delta waves. These are interspersed with some smaller and faster waves. As we reach stage 4 of non-REM sleep we have almost exclusive delta waves. Stages 3 and 4 are most often referred to jointly as slow wave sleep, and are considered deep sleep. It is often difficult to wake people out of stages 3 and 4, slow wave sleep. People who sleep through alarm clocks or loud noises are in this deep, slow wave, sleep cycle.

Oxygen intake decreases significantly during this stage, cortisol production ceases, and growth hormone is being released. Growth hormone allows the body to heal and aids in metabolizing fats. Slow wave sleep also is critical in declarative memory consolidation and in the regulation of the immune system. When we do wake from one of these deep sleep cycles we are groggy and disoriented because the brain waves are the slowest during these stages and furthest removed from the brain wave patterns of wakefulness. Have you ever noticed that sometimes when you wake up you are more alert and sometimes you are really groggy? This is because of the cycle you were experiencing when you were awakened. Awakening from slow wave sleep makes us feel sluggish. It is sometimes referred to as sleep inertia.

REM sleep is completely different from these first four stages. During REM sleep we expend a great deal of energy. Blood flow to the brain increases up to fifty percent more than it is during wakefulness. The term itself, REM sleep, is short for rapid eye movement sleep. Our eyes are very active during REM sleep, even though our eyelids may be closed. This is indicative of the fact that the brain is working. Certain neurons in the brain stem are particularly active during REM sleep. The neocortex, the thinking part of the brain is not as active, but the rest of the brain is basically processing experience, sensation, and information. Theta waves are emanating from the hippocampus supporting long-term memory consolidation (Mednick 2006, 42).

Additionally, the release of certain neurotransmitters is shut down during REM sleep, and as a result we cannot move our major muscles. We experience muscle paralysis (Martin 2002, 100–1). It is also during REM sleep that we have most of our dreams. The topic of REM sleep will be discussed in much more depth in chapter 4.

The point here is that once we achieve sleep, we go through these stages of non-REM sleep and then REM sleep, and this cycle takes about ninety minutes for an adult. For a newborn infant the cycle is only about sixty minutes and it gradually increases to about ninety (Martin 2002, 103). This is one cycle. It is interesting that these ninety-minute cycles are also present in our waking hours although they are less detectible. The waking cycle is called the ultradian rhythm (Martin 2002, 104). At night, however, we repeat these cycles all night long, every ninety minutes, unless we are awakened and sleep is disrupted. This means that if we sleep for eight hours, and our sleep is not disrupted by awakening or certain other issues that will be discussed, we will go through four or five cycles of sleep.

The time spent in these different stages also shifts during the night. We tend to spend more time in REM sleep during the later half of our night, while we get more slow wave sleep (stage 3 and 4) during the early part of the evening. Slow wave sleep is critical to our health. Consequently slow wave sleep will take precedence. Only when the need for slow wave sleep has been sated will we be allowed to spend more time in REM sleep. REM sleep is critical in the processing of experiences into memory and especially emotional memory. Hence if we don't get enough REM sleep we are prone to emotional or psychological problems.

Many people, unfortunately, consider sleep as wasted time. They think of it as a necessity only after they get done all that they want to do during the day. They will sacrifice sleep to go party. This is especially true of adolescents and people in their early twenties. How much sleep can they get by on? Well, the fact is this . . . sleep is crucial . . . it is critical . . . it impacts our health, our well-being, our mental functioning, our memory, our behavior, our productivity, and more. Adults really need about seven to eight hours of sleep a night, but most of us get far less than that. Children between ages five to thirteen need about ten to eleven hours of sleep, and adolescents need about nine hours (Mednick 2006, 78–79). How many adolescents do you know who are getting anywhere near nine hours of sleep a night?

One measure of whether we are getting enough sleep is how much we sleep on weekends or when we finally take that vacation? We typically try to catch up on sleep at those times. That is a clue that we are not getting enough sleep the rest of the time. Look at adolescent behavior as an example. They tend to sleep in on the weekends, probably all morning if left to their own devices. That is a clear sign of sleep deprivation (Martin 2002, 235).

There have been interesting sleep deprivation studies done with animals. When animals are deprived of sleep they die (Linden 2007, 186). It varies a little with the age of some animals, but within five days to two and a half weeks, the animals will die. It isn't that some will die. It isn't that half will die, or that most will die. All of them will die. Total sleep deprivation is 100 percent fatal. If they are allowed to sleep they will often recover, but without sleep they will die.

We cannot run such experiments with humans, but there are situations we can look at. What happened to American troops captured during the Korean conflict? The term "brainwashing" was thrown around a great deal. Captured American soldiers denounced the United States and avowed Communism as the way of life. We now know that there was no "brainwashing," no permanent psychological altering of the way people think (Linden 2007, 185). It was merely sleep deprivation.

If any of us are deprived of sleep long enough we will admit to anything, confess anything, say anything just to be allowed to sleep. The American soldiers had no long term trauma or change in their thinking or core beliefs. Once they were allowed to sleep they thought just as they had thought before the confessions. They were not "turned" to communism, they were not "brainwashed" . . . they were merely succumbing to sleep deprivation.

We need sleep. We must have sleep. Our bodies will not function without sleep. This is why we will doze off at our desks in the early afternoon. This is why students fall asleep at their desks in school. This is why we will doze off at the wheel of a car driving down the highway at sixty miles an hour. These are clues that sleep is important. Our bodies are saying, "You will sleep!"

There is also the interesting fact that some of us seem to be night people and some morning people. Why is that? What is the difference? We all have an internal timekeeper in our brains. This is called the circadian clock (Linden 2007, 203). This circadian clock keeps us on a regular cycle of sleep and wakefulness. It does seem to rely on external cues, specifically light and darkness, to remain completely accurate. In the absence of such light and dark cues, it gradually gets out of its cycle and we gradually go to sleep later and later in the evening and remain asleep later and later in the morning.

There is an area in the brain called the suprachiasmatic nucleus (Linden 2007, 203), which is responsible for controlling our circadian rhythms. It is located within the hypothalamus. The hypothalamus is responsible for some key functions. Besides controlling the circadian rhythm, it is also responsible for managing body temperature, hunger, thirst, anger, and fatigue (Wikipedia, 2001). Its functioning is also affected by stress.

Think about adolescents you know. Adolescence is a stressful time for multiple reasons, and look at the sleep patterns. Is there a connection between sleep patterns, stress levels, and the circadian rhythms in adolescence? Adolescents seem to move toward being night people, as opposed to morning people, during this phase of their life. It is really not surprising. Their physiology and hormonal changes impact melatonin release, pushing them toward later sleep onset.

A study was done in Minnesota (Wahlstrom 2002, 3–4)) in which the school start time for teens was changed to an hour later than the start time for younger children. This simple change resulted in adolescents who were less sleepy during the day, less depressed, less likely to arrive late to school, and who accumulated fewer absences. These are all outcomes which schools should be very interested in achieving.

Morning people tend to have a circadian rhythm that is almost exactly at twenty-four hours in length (Martin 2002, 124). Night people tend to have a slightly longer circadian rhythm, which is why bedtime starts to inch toward later and later hours. This is what happens with adolescents. Night people are more likely to need the influence of daylight to help regulate their circadian rhythm, but with the advent of the light bulb, it is possible to impact the circadian rhythm artificially and hence disrupt what would be considered its normal functioning.

Not only do adolescents in our society have the right physiology to be night people, but they also have the opportunity. Television programming is on all night long, the Internet never shuts down, and text messaging makes it possible to stay in touch twenty-four/seven. The degree to which light can shift our internal circadian clock is limited to roughly an hour per day (Linden 2007, 204), making the shift to being a night person gradual.

As an aside, modern air travel allows us to traverse numerous time zones in a matter of hours. However, adjusting our biological clocks to this change in time zones becomes problematic. This is why we have jet lag. Since the circadian clock can only adjust about an hour per day, if we travel over three or four time zones, it will take three or four days for us to really feel right. This is very significant for children traveling with you. It is also harder for the circadian clock to adjust to shorter days than to longer days, which is why jet lag is more pronounced if we fly east than if we fly west (Martin 2002, 119). Additionally, there is no jet lag flying north or south because we are not changing time zones.

Some people will take melatonin supplements, which can be either natural or synthesized, as a means of combating jet lag or other sleep disturbances. Melatonin is naturally produced in our brains by the pineal gland, which is influenced by the suprachiasmatic nucleus in the hypothalamus (Linden 2007, 206). Melatonin is actually derived from serotonin, and is useful as an anti-oxidant and in boosting the immune system. However, it can also have a negative impact on growth as well as some other potential issues, and therefore should not automatically be given to children or adolescents as a supplement. Natural melatonin levels normally peak about three o'clock in the morning for those whose circadian clocks are in sync.

Roughly an hour before we awaken in the morning a hormone called adrenocorticotropic hormone (ACTH) begins to elevate (Martin 2002, 107). This signals some other aspects of waking, including a rise in body temperature. If we are in a healthy circadian rhythm we can have an impact on ACTH release.

There have been some studies done where people were asked to wake themselves at specific times (Martin 2002, 107). By putting that thought in their heads they were able to awaken around the desired time. If someone was asked to wake themselves at four o'clock in the morning, for example, what the researchers found was that somewhere around three o'clock ACTH levels began to rise in the subject and they would then awaken somewhere around four o'clock. These studies were done with healthy individuals who had regular circadian rhythms. I suspect that individuals who were sleep deprived or who had circadian rhythms that were out of sync would not be able to awaken themselves at specific times nearly as effectively. That would include adolescents.

Aging can also impact circadian rhythms. As we age we tend to sleep less. That is not because we need less sleep, but rather because our ability to sleep diminishes. As we age we tend to have more aches and pains that keep us awake or awaken us during the night. We also tend to require more bathroom visits, which interrupts sleep cycles. Additionally we tend to be on more medications, which can have numerous and multiple effects on our ability to sleep through the night. However, would improving the level of sleep we get in childhood and adolescence, as well as developing better sleep habits during those years, have an impact on the aging process? This has not been studied but I believe it might.

If we are going to help our children we need to understand sleep, the cycles of REM and non-REM sleep, and the circadian rhythms that impact how and when we sleep. Now we can move on to discuss some of the things that occur during these sleep cycles.

# Chapter 3

# Sleep and Health

## The Immune System,
## Sleep Apnea, ADHD. . .

*There is this story of the transcript between a U.S. naval ship and a Canadian maritime contact off the coast of Newfoundland one foggy, foggy night. The transcript went as follows;*

*U.S. Naval Ship: Please divert your course 15 degrees north to avoid a collision.*

*Canadians: Recommend you divert your course 15 degrees south to avoid collision.*

*U.S. Naval Ship: This is the captain of a U.S. Navy Ship; I say again divert your course.*

*Canadians: No, I say again, you divert your course.*

*U.S. Naval Ship: THIS IS THE AIRCRAFT CARRIER USS LINCOLN, THE SECOND LARGEST SHIP IN THE UNITED STATES' ATLANTIC FLEET. WE ARE ACCOMPANIED BY THREE DESTROYERS, THREE CRUISERS AND NUMEROUS SUPPORT VESSELS. I DEMAND THAT YOU CHANGE YOUR COURSE 15 DEGREES NORTH OR COUNTER MEASURES WILL BE TAKEN TO ENSURE THE SAFETY OF THIS VESSEL.*

*Canadians: We are a lighthouse. . .your call.*

*We can be very bullheaded about a lot of issues, including sleep. What we need to do is start looking at the facts and forget our posturing. . .especially when it comes to sleep.*

Spending an adequate amount of time sleeping is critical to our health and well-being. What we typically think about when we don't get enough sleep is that we are tired. There is evidence that during slow wave sleep the glucose levels in the glial cells in the brain are restored, hence replenishing the brain with energy (Griffin 2006, 174–75). Not getting enough sleep, however, can have some devastating effects on us far beyond merely feeling tired and groggy.

Sometimes we don't get enough sleep because of acute situations or events. That could be the result of spending half the night in the emergency room with a loved one, or taking a night flight from New York to London, or having your water pipes burst on a cold January evening and spending the evening cleaning up water damage, and so forth. We try to catch up on that sleep as soon as we can.

There is also the cumulative sleep deprivation that many of us experience. That comes from getting only six to seven hours of sleep a night (when we really need about eight hours, or even more for children and adolescents) over long periods of time. That cumulative sleep deprivation is what many people live with in industrialized countries, and it takes a tremendous toll. Can adults get by on only five to six hours of sleep a night? Yes they can, but later in life they will pay the price. Children and adolescents not only will pay that price later in life, but will also pay a huge price during their developmental years. Our educational system is also paying quite a hefty price.

What are the consequences of sleep deprivation? One very interesting consequence of acute sleep deprivation is the progressive decline in body temperature. Acute sleep deprivation disrupts the body's ability to maintain a set body temperature. For humans, that set temperature is 98.6 degrees.

An interesting sleep deprivation study was done with rats (Griffin 2006, 60–61). The rats lived in a colony with multiple rooms. One of the rooms was kept at a very high temperature. The rats that were not sleep deprived would venture into that room but very quickly leave because it was so warm it was uncomfortable for them. The rats that had been deprived of sleep for an extended period would go into that room and remain there. They would not leave. Their own bodies were not maintaining heat and this room was, therefore, comfortable for them. A set temperature for the body is important because it helps keep bacteria in check.

Sleep deprivation also causes a progressive rise in body metabolism. We burn fuel at a quicker rate in order to elevate body temperature. This makes us want to eat more. The rats in the study, if allowed, would eat more food in an attempt to elevate body temperature. How much of the childhood obesity in this country is the result of or at least exacerbated by sleep deprivation?

Another significant result of sleep deprivation is its impact on the immune system. Various aspects of the immune system are related to the circadian clock within each of us. Consequently, anything that significantly or continually disrupts sleep disrupts our circadian clock, and therefore disrupts our immune system. Because sleep deprivation has a critical impact on the immune system we become more susceptible to infections, viruses, and bacteria of all kinds. Severe sleep deprivation will certainly have this effect, but moderate sleep deprivation—the ongoing cumulative kind of sleep deprivation—will also have this effect.

Consider what happens in public schools in December just before the winter break. Kids get sick. Teachers get sick. Parents are sick. We tend to think there are just a lot of viruses going around. In reality, the main reason for these minor but unpleasant illnesses is that we are exhausted. Students and teachers are all sleep deprived from the constant grind and stress of the first semester, and it begins to catch up with us. Our immune systems are not functioning as effectively as they do when we are well rested, and we get sick. What do most of us do when the winter break does come? We try to get caught up on sleep. Look at your adolescent's behavior?

Under normal circumstances one of the immune system's responses to infection is to release chemicals known as interleukin-1 (Martin 2002, 81). This chemical induces sleep and produces a fever. It produces the fever by adjusting the brain's temperature control center elevating the temperature set point. Hence we feel sleepy and feverish when suffering from an infection. The resulting higher temperature, the fever, fights the bacteria, and the sleep strengthens the immune system response.

As mentioned earlier, total sleep deprivation is fatal. It is always fatal, not just some of the time. In fact, other than allowing the animal to sleep, nothing else can be done medically to save an animal that has been deprived of sleep. There is a very curious finding in the autopsies of animals that die from sleep deprivation. The autopsy shows that a certain bacterium, which is normally restricted to the digestive tract, has been allowed to leave the digestive tract and colonize other organs. Since the body's own temperature and immune system are not doing the job of killing these bacteria as they normally would upon leaving the digestive tract, these bacteria are allowed to roam through the body and colonize and destroy other body organs. The animal's own digestive bacteria kill the animal. There is a very interesting story related to this with humans from World War II. Paul Martin recounts this story in his book *Counting Sheep* (2002, 82–84). The Germans and Soviets were fighting over the city of Stalingrad. The Soviet commanders set on a strategy of making continual raids on the German lines every evening. They would shoot flares into the air signaling their imminent attack. Then they would send a small number of soldiers to attack some point in the German lines. The point was not to break through the lines, but to continually harass the Germans. In fact, sometimes when they shot off the flares, they did not attack . . . but the Germans always had to be ready. The Germans never knew where the attacks would come, so every soldier had to be awake and ready.

The Soviets also would play loudspeakers all night long piping in propaganda or just loud music. The Germans became exhausted. They could not sleep, and they were not as efficient or effective as soldiers. More than that, however, the health of the German soldiers began to deteriorate. There were always some soldiers who died of infectious diseases, but the rates became much higher. The Soviets referred to this as the "German sickness." At that time no one knew that sleep deprivation could cause severe health issues.

Ultimately there was a totally new phenomenon. Seemingly healthy German troops began to die, and for no apparent reason. The sleep deprivation was causing or furthering their exhaustion and stress. Their metabolic rates were also increased causing them to require more food, which, because of supply issues, was not available. The Soviet strategy was planned to exhaust the German troops and make them less efficient in battle, but the tremendous effect that sleep deprivation had on the health of the soldiers and on their mortality rates was not understood until much later.

Another interesting issue has very recently come to light. That concerns the reports coming out that "graveyard" shifts are a probable cause of cancer (Cheng 2007). Working at night disrupts our natural circadian rhythm, which, in turn, disrupts the natural levels of melatonin released. Melatonin is a natural sleep inducer. As a result these night shift workers tend to not sleep as much or as efficiently, and their immune systems are gradually impaired. With an impaired immune system, cancer cells are allowed to spread. Recent studies are suggesting that while working night shifts can cause cancer, constantly rotating from day shift to night shift and back is even worse. That really disrupts the circadian rhythm.

Another study showed that individuals who have worked the night shift for eleven years or more are twice as likely to develop heart disease. (Martin 2002, 163–64) Likewise, elderly people who are sleep deprived are more likely to suffer heart attacks (Martin 2002, 74).

Sleep deprivation also affects liver function. It elevates the fat and phosphorus levels circulating in the blood, and it alters thyroid hormone levels. Sleep deprivation can impact glucose metabolism. Individuals who have been restricted in their sleep levels for several nights in a row take roughly 40 percent longer than non-sleep restricted subjects to regulate blood sugar levels after a high carbohydrate meal (Martin 2002, 79).

There is cause to believe that obesity, which is a significant factor in industrialized countries, is often related to sleep deprivation (Martin 2002,

78). For one thing, lack of sleep can make us flabby and give us that pot-bellied look. Growth hormone is necessary to repair our muscles. When we work out we tear muscles, and growth hormone is required to repair those muscles, which is how we build muscle from working out. However, growth hormone is released during slow wave sleep. If we are continually sleep deprived we get less growth hormone, which means muscles are not repaired, which means that over time muscle will be systematically replaced with flab (Martin 2002, 68). Bodybuilders should understand that sleep is a very necessary part of their bodybuilding program.

Other recent studies have linked both weight gain and diabetes to lack of slow wave sleep (Scripps Howard News Service, 2008). Children, by age seven, who had an average of less than nine hours of sleep, were more likely to be overweight and have higher levels of body fat than those who slept nine hours.

We know that lower levels of sleep affect metabolism and suppress one's ability to regulate blood sugar. Insufficient sleep increases the risk of diabetes, increases the risk of being overweight, and has a negative impact on the immune system for children. Even three consecutive nights of disturbed sleep was enough to make the body less sensitive to insulin. The resulting decrease in insulin sensitivity is like gaining twenty to thirty pounds in weight. We may very well delay the onset of type 2 diabetes by giving attention to sleep issues and by increasing the quantity and quality of sleep.

Yet another issue with obesity is that obesity can cause sleep apnea. Anything that decreases the flow of oxygen through the upper air passage when we lie down can cause sleep apnea, and certainly extra deposits of fat will do this. The interesting thing is that not only does obesity increase the likelihood of sleep apnea, but sleep apnea can help cause obesity. Sleep apnea disrupts sleep, less sleep results in an increased metabolism in order to regulate body temperature, which means more hunger, which leads to eating more food, which leads to more weight gain (Martin 2002, 302). This can become a vicious cycle.

Since we have introduced the topic of sleep apnea, let's spend a little more time there. First of all, is snoring related to sleep apnea? Snoring and sleep apnea are not the same thing, although they are related. Snoring comes from restricted air flow in the upper air passage at night. Anything that restricts this air flow or relaxes the muscles in this area can cause snoring. Excessive alcohol, sedatives, obesity, colds, upper respiratory infections, allergies, sleeping on one's back, enlarged tonsils, a receding chin, or even REM sleep (this will be discussed in chapter 4) can cause snoring (Martin 2002, 296).

When air flow is restricted in the upper air passage there must be greater effort to pull air through. Hence the air travels faster through a smaller cavity causing the soft tissue of the upper airway to vibrate. This is snoring. Heavy snoring means there is severely restricted airflow which itself impairs cognitive performance, manual dexterity, attentiveness, and mental alertness. One study among medical students found that heavy snorers had lower exam scores and were more likely than nonsnorers to fail exams. Heavy snorers failed exams 42 percent of the time compared to only a 13 percent failure rate among the nonsnorers (Martin 2002, 295).

In many cases heavy snoring is a sign of sleep apnea, and heavy snorers should be made aware of this possibility. If your child or adolescent snores heavily and regularly, that is a sign that they are not getting the sleep they need and their learning, productivity, motivation, and achievement levels are probably suffering. It would be wise to have it checked out.

While snoring restricts airflow, sleep apnea stops air flow, and that is the major difference. With sleep apnea the sleeper actually stops breathing. The upper airway is so restricted that air is not flowing in, and the physiological alarm system triggers a partial awakening in order to allow the airways to reopen so the sleeper can breathe. The individual then takes in a resuscitative snort of oxygen (Martin 2002, 297).

The problems with this are multiple. First, because the individual must come partially awake in order to breathe, it means that the quantity and quality of slow wave sleep and REM sleep are being disrupted. It also means that this individual is getting less oxygen in his blood. With less oxygen there is more carbon monoxide and the blood is more acidic. That can trigger an abnormal heart rhythm (Martin 2002, 305). Less oxygen in the blood also means the heart has to work harder resulting in higher blood pressure and ultimately potential heart disease (Martin 2002, 295). That means a greater likelihood of heart attack or stroke. Heavy snoring can have these results too, but sleep apnea is definitely a culprit.

Episodes of breathing stoppage can occur more than a hundred times a night. The number of such episodes per hour is called the sleep apnea index. Anyone who has an index of more than ten such stoppages an hour would be diagnosed technically as having sleep apnea. It should be apparent that sleep apnea is not a fixed state, but rather it is on a continuum. An individual who has breathing stoppages might have enough of those occurrences on a night when they drink alcohol heavily to qualify on the sleep apnea index. If an individual is having regular periods of breathing stoppage at night, even if it is not to the level of being diagnosed with sleep apnea, it is worth dealing with.

Any pattern of half waking and gasping severely disrupts sleep, and the result of that quickly becomes one of cumulative sleep deprivation. Besides the impact that has on one's immune system and all the other health effects already mentioned, it also is related to depression in adults. Roughly 45 percent of sleep apnea sufferers scored high on depression rating scales (Martin 2002, 306). Many adolescents also suffer from depression, and many have sleep apnea. In children, one study found that there was an unusually high proportion of children with sleep apnea who were ranked in the bottom 10 percent of students in school performance (Martin 2002, 306).

One final issue is that sleep apnea makes us tired. Besides all of the ramifications that being tired has for us either on the job or at school, it also can cause us to doze off at the wheel while driving a vehicle. That has also become a significant risk to people in industrialized countries. Drivers who have been awake for twenty-one hours performed as badly as drivers with an alcohol level of .08, which is the legal limit for drunk driving in many states within the United States (Martin 2002, 65).

Being tired or sleepy accounts for more traffic deaths than does alcohol, and yet we have no laws about driving while tired. (Martin 2002, 38). It is estimated that about 10 percent of fatal car crashes are the result of going to sleep or nodding off at the wheel, while 50 percent of all fatal truck accidents are related to sleep deprivation. That does not count the near misses, just the fatalities (Martin 2002, 34).

The implementation of Daylight Savings Time can even have an impact on accidents. Setting our clocks ahead by one hour in the spring, meaning we lose one hour of sleep that night, results in a peak in the number of fatal automobile accidents on the day after the time change (Martin 2002, 36).

Besides the fact that sleep deprivation impairs our driving ability, it also appears to impair our ability to recognize that our driving performance has been impaired (Martin 2002, 66). Since we have already mentioned alcohol, it is also important to note that being tired and drinking alcohol are not mutually exclusive. While both can and do cause accidents and death, when we are tired and also drink alcohol we amplify the effects of each on our systems (Martin 2002, 66). We know statistically that a lot of adolescents drink alcohol. We also know that a lot of them are sleep deprived. How many teenage automobile fatalities are the result of that combination?

Let's shift gears and look at the effect sleep deprivation can have at different stages in life. First of all, babies will normally sleep fourteen to sixteen hours a day. However, this sleep is not achieved all at one time. It is spread out throughout the day and evening. This is not the pattern that most adults have for sleeping. Because adults tend to sleep mainly in one block of time, dealing with a baby becomes very tiring for the adults, and these adults invariably end up suffering from sleep deprivation. Any young parent will verify this.

For the first four to five months new parents will lose about two hours of sleep a night, then about an hour a night for the next few years. Additionally, the sleep they do get is often interrupted and not good quality sleep. That means they are getting less slow wave sleep and less REM sleep. The result is fatigue, overly emotional reactions to each other and to the baby, and generally poor decision making. In some cases this state of exhaustion leads to abuse or neglect of the infant. An exhausted parent and a crying baby or a demanding preschooler can be a bad mix (Martin 2002, 222–23).

In early childhood sleep problems are becoming a huge concern. More than one in five children between the ages of four and twelve experience difficulty falling to sleep, snoring, and/or daytime tiredness. This is not really surprising. In many homes sleep is considered a maintenance activity, there are no real set bedtimes, and sleep is something you do only when you are too tired to watch any more television. Staying up is looked on as a desirable part of adult life. It is looked on as freedom.

There is growing evidence that childhood sleepiness is fueling emotional and behavioral problems in our children. When we get tired as adults we tend to lack energy and become less active. Children, on the other hand, resist their fatigue by becoming more active . . . even hyperactive. This revving up, combined with their underlying weariness, interferes with their ability to pay attention and behave properly in the classroom. Tired children will often not look tired, but they become irritable, fidgety, inattentive, disruptive, and difficult to manage (Martin 2002, 230–31).

Studies have shown that children who sleep well have a more positive self image, are more motivated at school, are more receptive to teachers, are less bored, and are better able to control aggression (Martin 2002, 231). It is estimated that between 5 and 10 percent of children in the United States have ADHD. This percentage has grown significantly over the past several years. However, there is also growing evidence that some of this increase in ADHD diagnosis is really the result of sleep problems (Martin 2002, 232).

If we treated the sleep problems that some children have due to breathing related problems, and addressed the lack of sleep that some children are getting because of parenting issues, the number of ADHD referrals would decrease. It is estimated by some that roughly one-fourth of all ADHD children could be cured of their symptoms by treating them for sleep related breathing problems (Martin 2002, 233).

It is also interesting that many ADHD diagnosed children are treated with Ritalin. Ritalin is an amphetamine-like stimulant that disrupts sleep. While it may suppress a child's daytime behaviors, it further impacts his sleep issues and therefore may be furthering the problem by masking the symptoms (Martin 2002, 233).

ADHD children also tend to be more resistant to going to bed. They fight sleep and fight parents when being put to bed. Their relationships with their parents suffer. About one-third of all ADHD diagnosed children were found to be habitual snorers, compared to only one in ten non-ADHD children. Snoring is one sign of sleep related breathing disorders. Again, that disrupts both the quality and quantity of sleep and ends up causing multiple other issues for the growing/learning child.

As we move into adolescence what do we see? Teens tend to treat sleep as a last resort. It comes at the bottom of their list of priorities. Most teens will stay up watching television, talking on the phone to friends, partying, or just hanging out rather than go to sleep. They get just enough sleep to get by, but not enough sleep to really function at their peak. Many teens are irritable, moody, forgetful, sometimes irrational, and often overly emotional about issues. Then on weekends or holidays they will lie in bed all morning. It can sometimes be very tough dragging them out of bed. These are classic symptoms of sleep deprivation. Numerous studies have shown that sleep deprivation is widespread among adolescents (Martin 2002, 234).

The way adolescents think about sleep and the choices they make about sleep significantly impact their behaviors, their moods, their decision making, and their academic performance. One study with fourteen-year-olds found that if they were restricted to only five hours of sleep it impaired their verbal creativity, verbal fluency, and ability to learn abstract concepts. It also impaired their motivation levels (Martin 2002, 64). Even one night without sleep impairs our ability to think flexibly and creatively. We also know that being sleepy causes people to take more risks. Think about the risky decisions that many teenagers make. They make risky decisions about driving (especially about speed), about drugs, about who to be with, and about where to be. Sometimes these decisions are extremely risky.

What happens when we start to get older? While that end of the aging spectrum may not seem immediately relevant to youth, it is important to educate them about what is normal and natural, and what we can actually influence. The older we get the less sleep we tend to get. That means we get less REM sleep and less slow wave sleep. Many of the symptoms of aging are also the symptoms of sleep deprivation. Is it possible that some of the symptoms of aging could be avoided or at least alleviated if we addressed the sleep issues? Probably so. We know that prefrontal cortex functioning is impaired by sleep deprivation and by aging. Getting more sleep, better quality sleep, or taking short naps could improve prefrontal cortex functioning.

Since elderly people typically get less sleep, they get less slow wave sleep, and they have less growth hormone released. Growth hormone, as mentioned earlier, is released during slow wave sleep. Growth hormone is important early in life because insufficient amounts of growth hormone can stunt growth. However, growth hormone is also necessary in repairing our bodies. When we exercise or do a lot of yard work we tear muscles, and growth hormone is necessary in repairing those muscles. Without sufficient growth hormone the muscles don't recover as quickly, we lose muscle strength, our joints don't work as efficiently, etc. We also will have more aches and pains.

There was an interesting study done with university students. Two weeks of slow wave sleep deprivation caused these young, healthy individuals to have aches and pains throughout their bodies just like elderly people have (Griffin 2006, 188).

One final, related thought concerns fibromyalgia. There are many children and adolescents who suffer from fibromyalgia. The pain from fibromyalgia can be so debilitating that the individual cannot continue normal daily routines. Fibromyalgia is linked to sleep disorders. Most fibromyalgia sufferers have sleep apnea or some other detectible sleep disorder. While fibromyalgia is not completely understood, it is believed that these sleep disorders are not merely a symptom of fibromyalgia, but may also be a cause of the condition (Wikipedia, 2001).

Clearly, slow wave sleep deprivation can have a tremendously negative impact on the health and well-being of children, and that certainly will impact what goes on in the classroom. Having laid the foundation for what occurs during non-REM sleep, let's move on to thinking about REM sleep.

# Chapter 4

# Sleep and Memory
## *What Is Memory and How Is It Stored?*

*There was an elderly couple talking to a neighbor and telling him about a wonderful memory course they were taking. The neighbor asked the old man who was teaching the class. The old man thought for a moment, scratched his chin, shook his head, and looked up and down trying to remember.*

*Finally he said, "What is that pretty red flower . . . it has thorns on the stem?"*

*"You mean, rose?" replied the neighbor.*

*"Yes, that's it," he said turning to his wife. "Rose, can you remember the name of that instructor?"*

Memory is the subject of jokes, it is the key element in learning, it is a main subject of discussion for those of us who are getting older, and it is the source of trauma and heartbreak for those dealing with family members who suffer from Alzheimer's disease. But what is it we really know about memory? To discuss one of the key functions of sleep, specifically REM sleep, we need to understand a little about memory, and that means a little about how the brain functions.

What is the function of the neocortex, the thinking part of the brain? Is the neocortex a little computer? No, actually it is not a computer at all. In fact, the main functions of the neocortex include memory storage, memory retrieval, and making predictions based on those stored and retrieved memories (Hawkins 2004, 105). This is what I.Q. tests are all about . . . "A is to B as C is to what?"

Memory is also the basis of who we are. It is the basis of how we understand ourselves and how we understand others. It is the basis of all of our relationships with others. If you have ever had a loved one who was suffering from advanced stages of Alzheimer's you clealy understand that. The Alzheimer's patient does not remember you, their relationship with you, or even who they are. They do not know you, they do not trust you. . . you are a stranger. They often begin behaving in ways they never behaved before. They might start cursing or just wandering off because they do not remember who they were.

Not only is memory the key component of our relationships, it is also the key component of our learning. Consider the task of walking and learning to walk. Jeff Hawkins does a wonderful job of discussing this in his book *On Intelligence* (2004, 91). A toddler goes through all kinds of arm movements and leg movements and even falling in the learning of the skill of walking. Eventually he gets it.

When we walk down the street, however, since we have learned the process of walking, we are retrieving past memories of muscle movements, and we are predicting that our foot will hit the pavement with each step we take. We are good at it, until we find ourselves in a deep conversation with a friend and we step off a curb that we did not notice. We flounder, we stumble, we fall, and/or we twist an ankle. The problem was not that our muscles reacted incorrectly. The problem was that we predicted incorrectly. We predicted incorrectly because we did not notice the curb, but the fact is we predicted that our foot would hit the pavement and it did not do so when we expected it would.

Learning sports provides another example. Learning to catch a fly ball in softball or baseball is a matter of recalling past memories of fly balls and predicting where this one will fall based on those past memories. We are not computing this. Computers, to this point, cannot do this. . . they cannot catch a fly ball. Humans can learn to catch a fly ball not because we are computing it, but rather we are retrieving memories and making predictions based on those memories. If it were computation we would have little geniuses who were great outfielders early on in life. That does not happen because this is not a matter of computation; it is a matter of memory recall and prediction based on those memories.

If our brains did act like computers in computing information to catch a fly ball then Albert Einstein might not have developed the theory of relativity. He would have been busy playing center field for the New York Yankees.

Another task computers cannot do is that of recognizing animals in photos. You cannot show a computer photos of animals and ask the computer to recognize which ones are cats as opposed to dogs, foxes, and so forth. The human brain can look at such photos and state, "that is a cat, that is a dog, that is another cat," and so on. The human brain can even see a partial picture of a cat, a cat with it's head sticking out from behind a lamp post for example, and the brain will recognize it as a cat (because the brain can also predict that the rest of the cat's body is probably there). Computers cannot do that. The human brain can do that because, again, it is a matter of memory and prediction rather than computation.

The fact of the matter is, as Jeff Hawkins points out, the key functions of the neocortex are those of memory storage, memory retrieval, and making predictions from those memories. This is not just a function of the neocortex, it is the primary function.

So, with that in mind, what role does sleep play in memory? To answer that, to put it in perspective, it is important to look at the past. What is one of the key differences between warm-blooded and cold-blooded animals? The answer lies in the question itself.

Warm-blooded animals maintain a specific body temperature, while the temperature of a cold-blooded animal is whatever the environment happens to be. To some that may sound like a minimal thing, but in reality it is significant. Being warm-blooded requires a great deal of energy, up to five times the energy expenditure of cold-blooded creatures (Griffin 2006, 57). For a human being to maintain a temperature of 98.6 degrees (or other animals to maintain whatever their temperature set point is) our bodies spend a great deal of energy.

What this means is that we must take in a great deal of fuel on a regular basis, which means we must eat on a constant basis. Our bodies require a great deal of fuel to maintain this set body temperature. A snake, on the other hand, spends no energy maintaining a specific body temperature. Its temperature is whatever the environment happens to be. Consequently, a snake does not have to eat every day, or even every week. It eats, or swallows, its prey and it may not eat for another month depending on the size of that meal. The point is, the snake spends no energy maintaining a body temperature, and thus does not have to eat on a regular basis. It does not have to search for food as a regular daily routine.

Since all warm-blooded animals must have a constant and regular supply of food to function optimally, warm-blooded creatures must seek food as a regular part of their routine. In industrialized countries we tend to forget that because we don't think about seeking food as part of our routine. In third-world countries finding the next meal is a part of daily life, and for street people in the United States finding the next meal is part of the daily routine. Because warm-blooded animals must have food and seek food regularly, we must be purposeful about finding food. Plant eating animals must know where to roam for food, and meat-eating animals must know where to look for prey. Consequently, warm-blooded animals must also be more mobile, but being mobile also means they must be on the lookout for predators.

All of this requires the ability to think. Hence the development of the neocortex, the thinking part of the brain. All warm-blooded animals have a neocortex. Humans have a much more developed neocortex than other animals, but all warm-blooded animals have a neocortex. Cold-blooded animals do not have a neocortex. Reptiles have periods of slumber, which seem to correspond to the non-REM sleep in warm-blooded animals, and they have periods of activity. These periods of activity, however, are more similar to a warm-blooded animal's sleepwalking than the true wakefulness that we experience (Coturnix 2005). Is this because the reptile has no neocortex? Probably so.

If warm-blooded animals require a neocortex to think (which is what enables them to catch or find food) in order to help maintain a constant body temperature, then they must also have a means of remembering. It isn't just humans who have memories; all animals with a neocortex have memories. A dog, for example, remembers the smell of its master, but it also remembers the smell of others who come to visit occasionally and it greets them appropriately. A dog will great its master at the door and will then go find the tennis ball because it wants to play fetch and remembers doing that. Or it will go to the dog bowl because it is hungry and remembers that the dog bowl is where it will get food.

The question then becomes, how much memory can we keep in our working memory in the neocortex? How much can we keep at the tip of our fingers, so to speak, in our memory? The answer is very little.

What we must have is the ability to file experiences into long-term memory so that we can recall them when we need them. We can't keep everything at hand in our working memory because we would overload the neocortex very quickly. How many items can you keep in your mind on a mental grocery shopping list? Unless you have a strategy for remembering lists, it is probably very few.

So, how do we store things into long-term memory? This is where sleep and especially REM sleep comes into play. Cold-blooded animals do not experience REM sleep (Linden 2007, 194). REM sleep is found only in warm-blooded animals, and REM sleep is found in all warm-blooded animals.

One of the main functions of REM sleep is that of storing our experiences into long-term memory. It is not surprising that the main time for processing experience and learning into memory would be during sleep, because that is when we are most likely not being bombarded with additional information through our perceptions.

There are some different views and theories about the function of REM sleep and we will discuss some of those a little later, but there is convincing evidence that at least one of the functions of REM sleep has to do with memory storage and retrieval. Let's be clear, the act of learning is all about memory storage and retrieval, because learning involves remembering and then repeating tasks. However, the process of remembering, of storing things into memory, does not just happen. This is another reason sleep is so important for children and adolescents. During these early years of life the main task is that of learning. Ongoing sleep deprivation compromises a child's ability to achieve this necessary task.

This is also why pulling "all-nighters" studying for a test is really inefficient learning. After the "all-nighter" the student may have the material in his working memory, but long-term memory is being compromised.

Before going further let's discuss memory for just a moment. Memory is not just one thing. We talk about memory in phrases like good memory or bad memory, or our memories are short, etc. But memory encompasses a lot more than what we typically think of as memory. First, there is declarative memory and non-declarative memory (Martin 2002, 253).

Declarative memory refers to memory of factual knowledge or experience. It is termed declarative because we can consciously discuss or "declare" the facts or experiences we know or we have had. Non-declarative memory refers to things we learn to do, like skills or procedures. Non-declarative memories are those that come to us without conscious thought or recollection of them.

Declarative and non-declarative memories are further broken down into subsets. Semantic memory and episodic memory are types of declarative memory. Semantic memory refers to knowledge of facts that are independent of time and space. Most standard textbook learning falls under the category of semantic memory. It is also the easiest type of learning and therefore the easiest type of memory to forget.

Episodic memory refers to memories of specific moments in time and space. Episodic memories would include the stories we tell about the things that have happened to us. Telling jokes is an example of episodic memory. Some people are better at telling jokes than others. The difference is really not any specific ability, but rather the emphasis we put on memory. Those individuals who are good at joke telling tend to think of the joke in terms of episodes. They are using their episodic memory. People who are not good joke tellers are trying to remember the words or how the joke progresses. In other words, they are trying to remember the joke utilizing semantic memory. The difference is really the approach we take to remembering the joke. It is far easier to remember a joke as a story . . . as an episode.

Episodic memory is always easier to remember than semantic memory, and that is mostly due to the fact that we can put it in time and space. In other words we remember the time or the location of the episode or event. For example, if asked what you had for dinner two weeks ago on Friday night your response might be, "I have no idea." But if asked if you went out to eat that evening you might respond, "Oh, yes, we went to my favorite restaurant . . . and I had shrimp scampi, rice pilaf, a salad with bleu cheese dressing. . ." Remembering the location triggered the other memories about the episode.

Using our episodic memory is also a useful technique in remembering semantic memory. Taking a test is a good example. A student taking a test may not be able to remember the answer to a question, but if he can visualize the teacher standing at the blackboard when he discussed that topic, in other words remember the episode, then often that will be enough to trigger the semantic memory . . . the factual answer to the question.

Social workers can use basically this same strategy when interviewing clients or family members. Sometimes if you ask a parent to tell you the problems their child is having they cannot adequately put it into words. In other words, they cannot access semantic memory well enough to describe the problems. However, if you ask them to relate the story of the last time their child had difficulties, they can often do that. They can relate the episodes, the stories, the events, and through accessing those memories you can more clearly assess the problems.

Non-declarative memory consists of procedural memory and automatic memory. Procedural memory would include such things as learning to ride a bike, learning to walk, or learning to tie a tie. If you can tie a tie and were asked to describe to someone else how you tie that tie, could you do it? Could you put it into words? You probably could with some effort, but you would most likely have to think your way through the procedure, or visualize actually tying the tie in order to put the event into words. Wearing a tie to work is an event many men have experienced for decades, but telling someone else how to tie it requires thinking their way through the procedure.

Procedural memory also comes into play at times when we are driving to well-known places. Have you ever sat behind the wheel of your car on a Saturday morning intending to go one place, you have a lot on your mind, and suddenly you realize that you have pulled into the parking lot at your office instead? What happened was that your mind was on other things and your procedural memory took over and got you where you most often go. As embarrassing as that sometimes is, procedural memory does help us function without having to really think about everything we do.

Automatic memory refers to those things we have learned that become automatic recall. Examples would be counting to a hundred or reciting the alphabet. If you were asked how well you know the alphabet you would probably say you know it very well. If asked to recite the alphabet you could do so in a matter of a few seconds. Easy, right?

But, if you were asked to recite the alphabet starting from Z and going backwards, how long would it take you? Now that is a different story. We know the alphabet well, but we know it in only one direction. To recite it backwards requires thinking it through forwards.

Another example of automatic memory would be recalling the music tracks on your favorite CD. If you have a favorite music CD and were asked what song was on track seven, would you know? Possibly, but most probably not. If, however, track six was played for you, right at the end of that song you would then undoubtedly be able to relate what was coming next on track seven. Or have you ever been asked to verify your identity by giving the last four digits of your social security number? Most of us must quietly recite the first five digits before we can give the last four. These are all examples of automatic memory.

Emotional memory is the final type of memory, and that could fall under the category of declarative memory or non-declarative memory. Most emotional memory can be discussed (declarative) but some is on a gut level experience and is not easily accessible for discussion (non-declarative). Emotional memory can include experiences or episodes that have happened to us, but they are underscored in our memory by the emotion of the event. Consequently they are very strong memories. Think back to a time you were thoroughly embarrassed or humiliated. How strong is that memory? Most likely it is very strong and when you talk about it, it brings back emotional reactions.

Emotional memory can also at times be non-declarative. Sometimes an event is so horrific, so frightening, so traumatic, that it is recorded in our memory as a somatic, visceral, guttural, non-verbal episode. This can happen with infants before they have language to put with the memories. It can also happen with post-traumatic stress disorder patients, when the experience is so traumatic they cannot put it into words. It isn't that they are reluctant to talk about it; it is that they really cannot talk about the experience because it was not stored with any accompanying language.

Having discussed memory, we can now move on to discussing the storage of memory. One strong theory is that REM sleep aids in the processing of experiences and learning into memory. In fact, if an animal or human is deprived of REM sleep during the critical period after learning, the memory of that new learning is impaired (Martin 2002, 250–51). Experiments have also shown that deprivation of non-REM sleep can have negative effects on the consolidation of non-declarative memory, but not to the extent that REM deprivation has (Linden 2007, 200).

REM sleep, on the other hand, seems to interfere with the consolidation of rules, skills, procedures, and subconscious associations (which are all non-declarative memories) but not for the memories of facts and events (which are declarative memories) (Linden 2007, 197). In one experiment subjects were taught a skill, then some of those subjects were deprived of REM sleep and some were allowed to sleep. Those allowed to get REM sleep improved their performance of the skill after sleeping. Those deprived of REM sleep had a good memory of the training event itself, but did not show improvement in the skill.

There is still much that is not understood about how memory is consolidated and the role of sleep in this process. Certainly evidence for sleep dependent memory consolidation for procedural tasks is strong, but evidence for declarative memory consolidation is weaker except when emotions are involved. REM sleep does have an impact if the declarative memory is emotionally charged. At that point the hippocampus, part of the limbic system or the emotional center of the brain, is clearly involved.

Brain imaging studies show that after sleep there is a reorganization of the brain regions involved in the tasks learned, which indicates that sleep alters the strategy used by the brain and allows a more automatic execution of the task (Stickgold, 2005, 2–3). In one study Stickgold reports that subjects were given a skill to learn. They were allowed to practice that skill, and their performance level was routinely checked, until it appeared that they had reached a plateau level and that further practice was no longer showing an increase in performance. Then they were allowed to sleep. After sleeping their performance level improved significantly. The brain seems to reorganize the task and promotes better performance through such reorganization.

Other subjects practiced the skill during the morning. Once the plateau level was reached, rather than sleeping, they were allowed to go through their normal daily activities. They were again tested on their performance level before going to bed that night, and their performance level was still at the plateau level. After allowing them to sleep, their performance level again jumped. This shows that the gain in performance level was not due to mere time lapse, but directly related to sleep.

Yet other subjects, both in the morning and evening training sessions, were allowed to drink alcohol before sleeping. Alcohol, we know, disrupts REM sleep. These subjects were allowed to sleep but, because of the alcohol, did not get their normal REM sleep and their performance levels did not show any improvement after sleep. The conclusion is that REM sleep is vital for the brain to reorganize the learned task, thereby improving the subject's performance on that task. This also supports the fact that students who are regularly drinking alcohol or using drugs are disrupting REM sleep and thereby hampering the memory process.

In yet another study (Stickgold 2005, 5) subjects were given complex problems to solve and they were provided a procedure with which to solve them. Unknown to the subjects, there was a simpler means of solving the problems. Twelve hours after the initial procedures were taught some of the subjects had figured out that there was a simpler method, and they employed that method. The subjects that slept during the twelve hour interval were more than twice as likely to find that simpler solution. This was despite the fact that no one was even informed that there was a simpler solution to be found. In other words, they were not consciously looking for a simpler solution but found one anyway. This is a very sophisticated role for sleep in memory processing.

The ability of the brain to store memory through sleep can also be impacted in various ways. Damage to areas of the brain, for example, can disrupt or depress REM sleep. The popular movie that came out in 2004, *50 First Dates*, was about a woman who suffered memory loss because of damage to her hippocampus in an automobile accident. The plot revolved around a young woman who could remember the past but could not process any new experiences into memory.

Surprisingly, there are very real cases similar to that movie. One such case involved a young man with severe and continuous seizures from an accident at age seven (Eichenbaum 2004). Ultimately, in order to alleviate the seizures, his hippocampus was removed. As a result he could not process new information into memory. He could remember the past. He could also retain information in his working memory, which means he could remember what went on that day. He could have a conversation with someone, for example, or he could watch a ball game and discuss the game.

The following day, after he had slept, he would have no memory of yesterday's conversation or ball game. He could rewatch a tape of the game he saw yesterday and think it was a new game. His declarative memory was thus impaired, but not his procedural memory.

After the surgery he was taught to type. Every day he was asked if he had ever typed, and his response was that he had not. Then they would ask him to try typing. Each day he did, and he continued to get better at typing until he could type very well. However, he had no recollection of learning the skill of typing. Consequently, although he could eventually type (because he could learn procedural memory skills), he had no recollection that he could type. When asked if he could type he would respond that he could not, but when he tried he would be amazed that he could.

Exactly what happens in cases like this, exactly how sleep is impaired and so impairs the ability to process experience into memory is not understood. However, there is clear evidence that it is crucial. There is a lot more that must be learned.

Certain drugs also impact REM sleep. Some drugs used as antidepressants, such as monoamine oxidase (MAO) inhibitors completely suppress REM sleep yet they seem to not significantly impact memory (Vertes and

Eastman 2000, 867). Some of the modern antidepressants, like Prozac, cause a reduction in the amounts of REM sleep but don't completely suppress it.

The fact that antidepressants do not seem to impact some memory may be due to several factors. First of all declarative and non-declarative memory are not processed in the same manner. Non-REM sleep, as has already been stated, may play a larger role than REM sleep in processing declarative memory. Secondly, we do not completely understand the nature of the processes involved in memory. Memory storage and memory retrieval may be two very separate issues, yet many researchers tend to describe memory consolidation as one issue. Hence there is confusion. We will talk more about this momentarily.

Illegal drugs, such as marijuana, may also have a major role in suppressing REM sleep. We know that the canabinoids in marijuana are fat soluble and thus remain in the brain for long periods after use. The question that must then be asked is what does marijuana use do to memory consolidation? Is it possible that the learning problems that regular marijuana users display are related to REM sleep loss? Is it possible they can still learn declarative memory related facts, but less so processes and procedures (such as mathematics) which are non-declarative related memory?

Memory can also be altered or changed over time. One way it can be altered is by source misattribution. That means that while we retain the memory, we don't remember where we got the information. We think we got it from one place when in reality it came from a different source. Have you ever told a joke to the very person who originally told you that joke? That is an example of source misattribution. Another example has been when someone writes a song and actually thinks they wrote the melody when, in fact, they heard it somewhere else. There are certainly times when people intentionally plagiarize, but there are also times when they really thought they had created it. Unfortunately lawsuits have been filed in cases that were probably legitimate cases of source misattribution.

Another way that memory can be altered is through suggestibility. In one study subjects witnessed a supposed crime (Linden 2007, 125). The subjects were then shown the suspects one at a time. None of the suspects they were shown was actually the perpetrator, and all of the subjects correctly stated that none of the suspects shown was the perpetrator. However, when subjects were shown all the supposed suspects at one time and asked to pick out the perpetrator, 40 percent selected the individual who looked the most like the actual perpetrator. Further, when the subjects were told before they saw the line-up of suspects that several others had already identified one of these individuals as the perpetrator, 70 percent of the subjects then picked a suspect as the perpetrator.

Children are, not surprisingly, even more suggestible than adults. In the 1980s there were numerous reports of child abuse. Many preschool children, when interviewed, were stating that their teachers had abused them. This led a number of researchers to examine what was happening (Linden 2007, 126). The researchers found that preschool children and even many younger elementary children could be made to manufacture allegations of abuse against an adult they knew if asked leading and suggestive questions.

Many of these headline cases in the 1980s were ultimately dropped or overturned on appeal. This is not to say that there were not legitimate cases of child abuse in the 1980s; there were, but the way children were interviewed led to some reports that were not legitimate. Today Child Protection Service investigators are trained to not ask leading questions when they interview a child who has possibly been abused. For example, if a child has a black eye, they are trained to ask something like, "How did you get the black eye?" rather than asking, "Who gave you the black eye?" The second question is a leading and suggestive question.

Regardless of the problems we have with memory, our memory capacity must be large, and our memories must be somewhat durable (Linden 2007, 127). Our memories must be stored in such a way that they can be retrieved readily, but not too readily. . .we do not want our minds always cluttered with memories that continually flood back into our consciousness. Our memories must also be malleable. They must be subject to change and modification based on subsequent learning or subsequent experience.

Given these parameters, it is not surprising that we sometimes do not have the same recollection of an event as someone else. Have you ever been telling a story of some past event and another individual who was also there (often a spouse) corrects you or gives a somewhat different account of the event? Who is correct?

What happens when we have an experience is that what we perceived is ultimately stored in memory. Then we replay the event in our mind, and also replay it during our sleep, sometimes multiple times over the course of weeks or months. As we replay it, and as our sleeping mind reprocesses it, it changes. The puzzled look we saw becomes a scowl in our memory. The question that was asked of us becomes an accusation. The other individual is going through similar changes, and when we finally recount the story three or four years later we find that our recollection and the recollection of our spouse might be substantially different.

It seems there is much evidence that sleep in general and REM sleep in particular has a role in memory storage. While there is still much to be learned, there are researchers pursuing this. There are also researchers who do not agree that REM sleep is important in memory storage, and there are some different theories about the function of REM sleep. While there are different theories about the function of sleep and REM sleep, there is one fact that is clear. If nature makes us sleep away so much of our time, whether we want to or not, then sleep must play a crucial role in our lives. Let's briefly examine some of these other theories of REM sleep.

To begin with there are researchers who disagree that memory consolidation is related to REM sleep. One reason cited is that some drugs, such as the MAO inhibitors mentioned earlier, which are mainly used as antidepressants, block REM sleep but seem to not have an impact on memory (Linden 2007, 201). Again, as mentioned earlier, what we call memory involves both declarative and non-declarative memory. REM sleep seems to play a larger role in non-declarative memory consolidation, so the fact that MAO inhibitors do not seem to impact declarative memory is moot.

Another argument cites the fact that some individuals with damage to the brain have reduced REM sleep or no REM sleep and they also seem to have no memory impairment (Siegel 2001, 1058–63). Again, however, they are talking about declarative memory consolidation. It would be interesting to do some studies on such brain-damaged individuals and test non-declarative memory impact and/or emotional memory impact.

Some researchers have also pointed out that studies with rats that inhibit REM sleep are also creating stress in rats, and that it may be the stress that is interfering with learning (memory consolidation) rather than the lack of REM sleep (Siegel 2001, 1058–63). That is a good point. How can you inhibit REM sleep in a rat and not induce a certain level of stress? However, there have been sufficient studies with humans that demonstrate the learning–REM sleep connection. These studies are always with subjects who volunteer and know what is happening so the stress level is minimized.

Another issue sometimes cited is that there are differences in the amounts of REM sleep among animals. Carnivores get the most sleep, herbivores the least, and omnivores (including humans) are somewhere in the middle (Marshall 2007, 6). Some researchers state that this is because animals have learned through evolution that there is no need to waste energy after they have eaten and don't need more food. Hence a large carnivore, like a lion, that has recently eaten will sleep more because it does not need to go searching for more food for a period of time.

Could there be another explanation? Is it possible that carnivores get more sleep because they in fact require more REM sleep? Could it be that the hunt, the chase, the kill require more REM processing than finding some grass to munch on?

During the cave man era of human development the cave men were typically the hunters and cave women were typically the gatherers. While gathering nuts, berries and other foods would require a certain amount of REM sleep to process into memory, the hunt was the topic of stories around the campfire. These events would certainly be the stuff of dreams (the processing of emotional experiences) for weeks or months afterwards. Would it not be the same for all animals? Carnivores would have a much greater need to process the emotional experience of the hunt than would herbivores in processing the grass or roots they found that did not run or fight back.

Another study (Siegel 2001, 1058–63) had subjects learn a skill and then let them sleep. When they entered a state of REM sleep they were awakened and asked what they were dreaming about. Only a small percentage were dreaming about the learning task they had undergone. Therefore, it was determined that REM sleep did not play a significant role in learning the task.

First of all, we have cycles in our sleep, and we go through a full cycle every ninety minutes. That means in every ninety-minute cycle we have gone through another cycle of REM sleep. Additionally, the REM stages of sleep tend to be longest during the second half of our eight-hour (optimally) night of sleep. Consequently, unless these subjects were awakened during every stage of REM sleep all night long how would the researchers know that the training was not a part of REM sleep that night? There is simply no way they could know that.

Secondly, if they were waking subjects from REM sleep, then they were interrupting the REM cycle, and hence interfering with the content of the subjects REM sleep. In other words, the subject might have dreamt about the training if they had not been awakened.

Thirdly, during a REM sleep period we have multiple dreams about multiple experiences and events. Just because the subject was not dreaming about the training at the exact moment they were awakened does not mean that they would not or did not dream about it in another part of that particular REM sleep period. To conclude that REM sleep is not a necessary part of memory consolidation based on this study is incredibly presumptuous.

Another theory of the function of REM sleep is that REM sleep promotes the development of the brain itself (Martin 2002, 246). When there is a lack of stimulation, as when the fetus is in utero, REM sleep provides the necessary stimulation for development. That is why infants spend more time in REM sleep than adults. This theory concludes that REM sleep is correlated to immaturity at birth. Animals that are more immature at birth do require more REM sleep. Human babies require a great deal of REM sleep. The amount of REM sleep always diminishes as animals move into adulthood.

One such study (Siegel 2005, 1269) cited that light deprivation to a developing eye in animals caused damage to that eye. When REM sleep deprivation was also linked to the light deprivation, the damage to the eye was more severe. All of this information supports the idea that REM sleep is important in brain development.

Playing devil's advocate, however, if this were the only function of REM sleep why does REM sleep continue to be a requirement for us into and all through adulthood? Secondly, what is brain development anyway? In the case of the light deprivation to the eye, is it not true that what is really happening is the forging of neural pathways from the eye to the vision areas in the brain? With light deprivation, the brain is assuming the eye is dysfunctional and does not waste the effort to forge neural pathways (Greenfield 1997, 114).

On the other hand, what is learning? When we learn, the brain forges neural pathways and actually changes as we learn with stronger neural pathways and bushier dendrites. Hence, brain development and learning (memory) are very similar processes at worst, and therefore the idea that REM sleep is necessary for brain development is not at all exclusive of the fact that REM sleep is necessary for learning and memory.

Another theory is that REM sleep is necessary to eliminate undesirable modes of electrical activity in the brain (Martin 2002, 247). Basically this is the opposite of learning. The brain is susceptible to overload and must be cleansed or purged of the unnecessary information. The idea relies on the thinking that memories are stored over sets of synapses and this is why we have such an associative aspect of memory. . .why one memory leads to another memory and so forth.

Since memories are stored in overlapping synapses, and since each synapse contains multiple different memories, these must be purged regularly to not overload the brain. The thinking is that REM sleep, and therefore dreams, are all about the information we are purging or trying to erase from memory. There are significant holes in this theory. First of all, is the material covered in dreams that which our brains are trying to forget? Not really. Secondly, sometimes after we dream we find that we have solved significant issues. We will discuss much more on dreams in a later chapter, but the reverse learning theory does not seem to stand up to close scrutiny.

What really happens with memory? This is really such a new area that there is still much to be learned. There have been many researchers studying sleep and many researchers studying memory, but until 1994 these two areas of interest were studied independently. It was not until 1994, just a little over a dozen years ago, that a paper came out linking the two (Stickgold 2005, 1272). The understanding that sleep is critical in memory consolidation is like a new frontier to be explored. Consequently there have been different theories emerging because we don't yet know enough of the facts.

We have already discussed the fact that memory is classified as either declarative or non-declarative, but in another dimension memory is also classified by duration. We have what is called working memory, short-term memory, and long-term memory. Working memory is the most transient. That is the memory we have while we are having a conversation. It keeps us from repeating ourselves and it allows us to follow a line of thought or a story. Working memory comes into play when we hear a phone number and try to write it down before we forget it. Dopamine is a neurotransmitter that functions in tuning the thought spikes during working memory (Linden 2007, 119). That is why people with Parkinson's disease or schizophrenia, conditions which are associated with dopamine irregularities, have trouble on tasks requiring working memory.

Short-term memory comes next in duration. Memories are initially stored in the hippocampus, and can be stored there for one or two years. This is short-term memory. Ultimately we know that memories are transported to other locations. Visual memories are ultimately stored in the vision centers of the brain while auditory memories are stored in the auditory areas and so forth. This is long-term memory.

The fact that memories are ultimately stored in the perceptual areas where they were originally perceived is an interesting aspect of memory. The sights one had at a birthday party are stored in the visual areas of the brain. The sounds from that party are stored in the auditory areas. The taste of the cake is stored elsewhere, and so forth.

Have you ever had the experience of remembering a conversation with someone. . .you can visualize the person's face, you can visualize the way they were moving their hands and their facial expressions, but you cannot remember what it was you were talking about? That is because the visual memories and the auditory memories of that conversation are stored in different locations.

The triggering of one aspect of the event is often enough to trigger all of those related memories, but not always. Sometimes the triggering of one aspect will bring back the other parts of a memory. As mentioned before, a student taking a test may not be able to remember the answer to that test question, but if he can visualize the teacher standing at the blackboard while he was explaining that subject, then the visual memory can sometimes trigger other memories and the student can come up with the answer. This is why bringing as many of the senses into play as possible during the education process will aid a child in the learning process.

So what is the difference between short-term and long-term memory? Is it that memory for facts and events are stored in the hippocampus for up to two years and then moved to long-term memory, or is there something else going on? Is it possible that memories are stored both in the hippocampus and, through aspects of both REM and non-REM sleep, are moved to long-term memory at the same time?

Is it possible that retaining these memories in the hippocampus is what allows us, again through sleep, to strengthen these memories for memory retrieval from long-term memory? After all, we know that as we learn, neural pathways are strengthened and dendrites are grown and become bushier in appearance as the learning solidifies. This allows for easier recall of the learning, but it does not happen overnight. It takes time to develop and strengthen these neural pathways and dendrite projections.

Here is what possibly occurs. Events, experiences, or factual information are perceived and processed into memory through sleep. It is processed into short-term memory and transferred to long-term memory storage areas through aspects of REM and non-REM sleep. It is retained in the hippocampus, in short-term memory, until those memories are either solidified as important to us or not reinforced because they are not important. Those that are important are reinforced in our sleep.

When we have important, significant, or emotional experiences in our lives we do not think about these events once and then forget them. We mull them over in our thoughts, and therefore in our sleep, over and over and over again. An emotional experience is one that stays with us for a long time. We think about it, we worry about it, we rehash it in our thoughts, we brood over it, we may cry over it. This may go on for weeks, months, or sometimes (as with grieving) for years.

Our dreams are a representation of those issues that are going on in our lives and in our thoughts. Hence, when we have experiences in our thoughts for long periods of time, they are also the stuff of our dreams for long periods of time. Hence they are underlined, bolded, italicized in our memories. The neural pathways involved in those memories are strong and bushy. Events that occur that we do not replay in our minds are not so reinforced and are therefore not at all easily retrievable.

The suggestion is that memory storage and memory retrieval are separate parts of the process and that we store memories fairly easily, but that the process of forging strong and lasting neural pathways for memory retrieval is what takes time. That is really memory consolidation. We don't understand memory well because it has these different components, and these require the cycling of sleep. REM sleep, slow wave sleep, and stage 2 of non-REM sleep are all somewhat implicated in sleep-dependent memory. These components require both REM and non-REM sleep to ensure proper memory storage and memory retrieval.

What about accidents and brain trauma? Some individuals with brain trauma have lost the last year or two of their memories. They can remember past events in their lives prior to the accident, but they cannot remember the accident or anything that occurred the year or so before the accident. That period of time just seems to be gone, and cannot be retrieved. Is it that those memories are really gone? Could they be retrieved? Is it the retrieval of memories that has been damaged and not the fact that the memories themselves are lost?

There has been research done during open brain surgery. The brain has no nerve endings and cannot feel pain; therefore surgery that is done on the brain can be done while the patient is awake so that they can respond to questions. Electrically stimulating specific areas of the brain during such surgery can result in the patient having very vivid memories of past events. Is it possible that, in cases where individuals have lost a year or so of their recent memory because of brain damage, these individuals could retrieve a memory from that period if we could electrically stimulate the exact areas where that memory was stored? That would shed light on whether the memory was lost or whether just the ability to retrieve that memory was lost.

It is frustrating that as of yet we know so little about the relationship between memory and sleep, but it is also exciting that there is so much we have yet to learn. While we don't yet understand the process thoroughly, we do know for certain that sleep is a crucial piece of the process of memory and learning. That means sleep must be understood as a crucial element in the lives of children and adolescents, and as a crucial element in their education. For memory to be retrievable long term requires proper amounts of sleep. There is a difference between learning something short term for test taking, versus learning it long term. . .for life. What are our educational goals?

# Chapter 5

# Functions of REM Sleep

## REM Sleep and Depression, Schizophrenia, Bipolar Disorder

*What is the difference between a painter and an eye doctor? The most significant difference may be in what they want us to see. They eye doctor wants us to see the world as it is. The painter wants us to see the world as he sees it. In truth, however, is there really a world "as it is," a world that we all see the same? Is there one reality? Or is it that we all see our worlds through different lenses? That for each and every one of us the world we know is the one that we have built based on our different perceptions and colored by all of our past experiences and our past perceptions?*

*If that is so, then we all must in reality see the world differently. We must all see the world as a painter. Truly communicating with other people is not about trying to get each other to see "a" reality, but rather trying to truly see what the other person sees and trying to help them see what we see.*

REM sleep is a critical part of the sleep experience. There are some specific issues that are related to this part of the sleep cycle. One of these is that our antigravity muscles are impaired during REM sleep creating a muscle paralysis. Some people, upon waking up, have experienced a very temporary paralysis. They cannot move. This paralysis is very brief, but undoubtedly frightening the first time it happens to someone.

When it does occur it is because the individual awoke suddenly from a REM sleep state and the muscle paralysis of that state had not yet subsided. It is nothing to worry about. This muscle paralysis is a normal part of REM sleep for humans and all other animals that experience REM sleep. In other words, all warm-blooded animals experience this REM sleep muscle paralysis.

Why do we experience a muscle paralysis during REM sleep? The reason is simply that it protects us. It is a safety mechanism. Our motor cortex is working during REM sleep and all the brain mechanisms necessary for movement are working quite well during REM sleep, but in our brain stem communication between the brain and the skeletal muscles is actively inhibited. The brain is very active during REM sleep. We have multiple dreams during this state. If it were not for this communication inhibition we would act out those dreams, and we could easily be hurt.

Michael Jouvet did some interesting research with cats along this line (Martin 2002, 101). He created a lesion in the brain stem, which in effect stopped the inhibition of communication between the brain and the muscles. What occurred was that these cats acted out their dreams. They stalked imaginary prey, they pounced, and they ate imaginary prey. They did this while real food was right at hand. The point is, acting out our dreams can be very dangerous. For humans it could mean walking into walls, walking out into the street, jumping out windows, and so forth. For animals it could result in being eaten by a predator because the animal is responding to a dream world rather than the real world.

There are in fact individuals who suffer from a condition called REM sleep behavior disorder. In this disorder the muscle paralysis does not exist and these individuals get up and act out their REM dreams. Since dreams can be scary and violent, the resulting behavior that is acted out can be, and often is, scary and violent. Individuals with this disorder have beaten up their sleeping partners and often injured themselves, sometimes quite seriously.

REM sleep behavior disorder, referred to as RBD, should not be confused with sleepwalking. Typical sleepwalking occurs during non-REM sleep. While most dreams occur during REM sleep, some do occur during non-REM stages, and this is typically when someone will sleepwalk. While some adults sleepwalk, most have grown out of doing so. Sleepwalking is most common between the ages of eight to twelve. Precautions should be taken so that sleepwalking children do not injure themselves, but other interventions are usually not necessary. Dreams that occur during non-REM sleep are typically not as bizarre, scary, or violent as REM dreams. This is because it is during REM sleep that we are processing the emotional experiences and thoughts.

An interesting aside of REM muscle paralysis is that people who are hypnotized often experience the muscle paralysis of REM sleep. When they come out of the hypnotic trance they often express feeling that their body felt so heavy it was stuck to the chair (Griffin 2006,190). Another effect of REM sleep muscle paralysis comes in the form of snoring. Because of this muscle paralysis the muscles of the throat sag, which creates a smaller upper air passageway, and can result in snoring. Some individuals who snore do not snore all night long, but rather just during the stages of REM sleep.

Another impact of REM sleep concerns depression. A depressed individual typically gets too much REM sleep (Martin 2002, 64). During REM sleep the mind is very active, as signified by the fact that the eyes are moving rapidly under the eyelids. During the phasic component of REM sleep we have a discharge of PGO spikes. These are part of an alerting or orientation response. During waking states this orientation response would make us turn toward a loud noise, a sudden motion, or anything new or novel in our environment. The excessive firing of these PGO spikes during REM sleep, which results from the processing of experience into memory and the dreaming that accompanies it, is exhausting.

Individuals suffering from chronic depression have a great deal of stress in their lives. There are issues that they worry about but may not do anything about, other than worry. The worries are constant. During REM sleep we are processing experiences, and spend a great deal of time processing emotional experiences into memory. Since depressed individuals have a great deal of emotional "stuff" to process they spend a lot of time in REM sleep. Because REM sleep is exhausting, these individuals wake up from sleep exhausted. Because they are exhausted, and exhaustion certainly effects motivation to act, these individuals have no energy to focus toward those issues that they are worrying about. This becomes a vicious cycle, and they remain in this state of depression.

Treatment for depression often involves antidepressant drugs like Prozac. Prozac will inhibit the uptake of serotonin, a neurotransmitter that soothes or calms us, and it also regulates the amount of REM sleep (Linden 2007, 201). Some of the older antidepressants completely stopped REM sleep. Prozac does not stop REM sleep, but it does decrease the amount of REM sleep that an individual gets. Partial sleep deprivation, which can be accomplished by waking the depressed individual about halfway through their sleep cycle, can also be effective with some individuals because it temporarily eases their depression.

Prozac and/or using partial sleep deprivation are useful tools to assist in helping depression in adults, but antidepressants may increase suicidal thoughts in children and adolescents. The benefits of using antidepressants with children or adolescents must be carefully weighed against the risks. Regardless of age, depressed individuals need some therapy to address the stressors in their life. They need to talk through those issues that are causing the stress and worry, and find and execute strategies to alleviate those stress-causing issues. Teens who are depressed need to work through and talk through their depression. Unless they do that the benefits of any other treatment will be minimal.

The fact that depressed individuals get more REM sleep has another impact. Because they are spending more of their sleep time in REM, they are spending less time in slow wave sleep. A lack of slow wave sleep dampens the immune system thereby making depressed individuals more susceptible to colds and viruses. It also undoubtedly makes them more susceptible to more serious consequences such as cancer or diabetes.

Additionally, as mentioned earlier, it is during slow wave sleep that growth hormone is released. Growth hormone not only stimulates growth in childhood, but has multiple other functions (Wikipedia 2001). Basically growth hormone repairs the damage we do to our bodies during daily living. Because depressed people spend less time in slow wave sleep, and hence have less growth hormone released, they tend to have more aches and pains throughout their bodies. This also acts to decrease motivation. It is hard to get motivated to attack your problems when you hurt all over.

Another question involves the relationship between REM sleep and major psychoses. There seems to be no clear or universally accepted understanding of the reasons for so-called psychotic breakdowns. However, they are most often preceded by extreme stress, extreme anxiety, major depression, or sometimes the use of mood altering drugs (Griffin 2006, 189) . . . all of which are common in the adolescent world.

We also know that all the major psychiatric disorders, such as schizophrenia, bipolar disorder, and major depression have associated sleep disturbances. Sleep disturbances have been noted as symptoms of these psychiatric disorders, but until recently had not been considered as possible contributors to these disorders. Is it possible that the sleep disturbances, especially the REM sleep disturbances, are in fact a contributing factor in these disorders?

Some studies have demonstrated that people with schizophrenia have difficulty with some simple procedural learning tasks, which is a function related to sleep-dependent memory consolidation (Stickgold 2005, 1275). Additionally, chronic schizophrenic patients will show improvements in certain learned finger tapping tasks after practicing such tasks, but they demonstrate no overnight improvement as would be expected following REM sleep (Stickgold 2005, 1275). At least some of the issues schizophrenia patients demonstrate are related to sleep dysfunction. How many adolescent schizophrenic patients could be helped merely by addressing their sleep disorders?

Linden points out (2007, 215) that portions of the prefrontal cortex are deactivated during REM sleep. The prefrontal cortex is critical in executive function, in other words in such tasks as judgment, logic, and planning. It is also important in working memory. The deactivation of the prefrontal cortex during REM sleep may be why REM dreams are often illogical, and why the individual having the dream willingly accepts the illogical, bizarre nature of the dreams.

This could also be why there is a hallucinatory property to REM dreams. It is interesting that the disconnection of the prefrontal cortex is also a hallmark of hallucinating schizophrenics. The hallucinations that a schizophrenic patient has are dreamlike experiences that are occurring during waking hours.

Is it possible that this is what schizophrenia is really all about? Is it that the world of the schizophrenia patient is one where their reality is being processed through a REM sleep state of mind (Griffin 2006, 191)? We know that when individuals face a great deal of stress and worry, as in depression, they require more REM sleep to process the stress and worry that they are experiencing. Is it possible that schizophrenic patients are so overloaded with stress, worry, or anxiety that ultimately they cannot take the strain? Is it possible that their ability to separate the world of reality from the world of REM sleep becomes impaired (Griffin 2006, 191), and that they end up responding to REM-like experiences during their waking hours?

A study by Kojima noted that a decreased ability related to the perception of motion often accompanies schizophrenia (Winstead 2001). In fact, the study showed that visual testing can be a reliable marker in determining schizophrenia. A study by Rybakowski found that most schizophrenic patients did have some degree of eye-movement disturbance (Winstead 2001). Some of the eye-tracking disturbances occurred when smooth eye-tracking movements were interrupted by rapid eye movements.

Earlier we discussed the fact that PGO waves, which accompany rapid eye movement during REM sleep, are a part of the orienting response during waking. In other words, it is what draws us to look at a sudden motion or turn to a loud noise. Is it possible that the eye movement, eye-tracking disturbances experienced by schizophrenics are the result of "experiencing" something that is not there during the slow eye-tracking task? That their waking world is disrupted by REM sleep, hallucinatory, experiences?

Another disorder known as catatonia, which is often but not exclusively associated with schizophrenia, could also be related to REM sleep. Patients suffering from catatonia may experience severe motor immobility in which their body and limbs seem to be locked in a pose for long periods of time. Earlier in this chapter we discussed the muscle paralysis that accompanies REM sleep. These seem to be similar states. Is it possible that in some cases of catatonia it is the REM state of muscle paralysis that is spilling over into the patient's waking hours (Griffin 2006, 192)?

The answers to these questions are not yet known, but it will be inter-esting to understand the relationship between REM sleep and schizophre-nia more fully, as that may lead to better interventions to help those who suffer from this disorder. If we can intervene effectively in the early onset of this disorder—in the adolescent years—we may make the lives of some schizophrenic patients more bearable.

*Chapter 6*

# Dreams and REM Sleep

## *What Are Dreams and Why Do We Have Them?*

*The maintenance manager of a large, forty story hotel in New York City hired a new employee. The employee was a country boy who had just moved to the big city and the manager wanted to give him a break. He instructed the employee to clean the elevators and then come back to see him for further instructions. By the end of the day the new employee had still not returned and the manager thought the man had decided not to take the job after all. Three days later the new employee turned up, much to the manager's surprise.*

*"Where have you been?" queried the manager.*

*"I've been cleaning the elevators," said the employee. "It was a big job. There are forty floors in this building and two elevators on each floor. And sometimes they aren't even there."*

*Dreams can give us that elevator experience . . . they can be very confusing.*

There has been a lot of thinking, a lot of discussion, a lot of writing, and a lot of disagreement about dreams, the function of dreams, and the meaning of dreams. Freud did a lot of thinking and writing about dreams. A good part of his career revolved around the meaning of dreams and dream interpretation.

There is a mystical air about dreams. Dreams have been interpreted as religious experiences or as warnings about the future. Dreams have been interpreted as glimpses into other worlds. Dreams have been looked on as insightful, as a means to reveal our innermost thoughts and drives, and therefore as a means of understanding and coping with our problems.

Dreams can also be very disturbing. This is especially true for children and adolescents when they experience nightmares. What are dreams really all about? That is what we want to explore here.

Freud thought that dreams were incredibly important in understanding our behavior and motivations. His book, *The Interpretation of Dreams (1953)*, bears this out. In fact, his entire system of psychoanalysis is based on his dream theories. While his theories about dreams and their interpretation are not widely accepted today, they did have a major impact on psychology and psychoanalysis.

Some people theorize that dreams function as mood regulators (Linden 2007, 217). That dreams allow us to process emotions, especially negative emotions, and by doing so it allows us to wake up feeling better and more able to face what is in store for us the next day. Others think that dreams serve as a kind of psychotherapy (Linden 2007, 217) and that both psychotherapy and dreams allow the mind to make connections between life events in a safe and protected environment without being influenced by outside issues. Yet others think that dreaming has an evolutionary adaptive function, that dreams evolved as a time to rehearse and perfect behaviors that are necessary for our survival during our waking hours (Linden 2007, 217).

A relatively new theory is that dreams function to allow us to act out the undischarged emotional arousal from our unfulfilled expectations of the previous day (Griffin 2006, 33). This is referred to as expectation fulfillment theory. Paraphrased this theory states that:

- Dreams are our metaphors for emotionally arousing thoughts that are present at the onset of sleep.
- The expression of these emotionally arousing thoughts as a dream completes the emotional circuit and thereby deactivates the emotional charge. This is what frees the brain to deal with the emotionally arousing concerns of the next day.
- With this completion, by acting out through dreaming the previously unacted-out thoughts and emotional concerns, the emotional templates are cleared for use the next day (Griffin 2006, 36).

Yet another theory, and one that I personally think is the most supported by the data from recent studies, is that dreams are related to memory processing. That it is during our dreams that we cross-reference, integrate, reprocess, and consolidate memory (Linden 2007, 217).

Hobson, from Harvard University states that

the main purpose of cycling sleep is memory consolidation and integration, and that the experiences of narrative dreams are basically what the logically impaired and hyper-emotional brain can stitch together into a narrative from scraps of mostly visual memory. The content of dreams is merely a funhouse-mirror reflection of memory consolidation and there is no need for dream interpretation. (Linden 2007, 219)

In other words, dreams are basically a side effect of memory consolidation. Dreams are of no real importance and they have no real function. What is happening in our brains is that memories are being processed during REM sleep, and that dreams are the attempt by our minds to make some sense of the data that we are processing into memory. This helps explain why we don't remember dreams any better than we do. We have dreams all night long during our REM sleep states, and yet we recall very few of them. Typically the only ones we do recall are the dreams we were having when we were actually awakened, and those only stay with us briefly unless we write them down or make some effort to remember them.

This is what happens when children have nightmares. Children, who have very little real world experience to draw on, are processing their experiences during sleep. Because of their lack of knowledge and experience things are scarier for them in the first place (not to mention horror movies or movies that are not horror movies for adults but are for children), and the resulting dreams are so intense that they are awakened and remember the dreams.

Outside of nightmares, some people do seem to recall their dreams better than others, but if dreams really had more of a function in our lives, wouldn't we as a species have developed a better means of remembering them? Would we not have evolved some adaptive mechanism to better recall our dreams if they really were an important part of sleep?

Do dreams have meaning? Sure they do because we dream about the issues we are facing in our lives. Our mind is processing the learning and the experiences of the most recent waking period, cross-referencing those with past events by bringing up our past related memories, and making the effort to store these recent experiences in relation to past experiences.

Have you ever stood and watched someone making a pizza? Certain pizza parlors even have windows where kids can watch the pizza chef throwing the pizza dough into the air and preparing it for the oven. Dreaming is like watching pizza being made. The important work is the making of the pizza. Our mind is processing experience into memory. The dream is like watching the pizza being made. It is interesting and exciting, but it is just a show. Our dreams are just a product of our brains watching, and in their own way interpreting, what is going on with the memory processing aspect of sleep.

Consequently, do we need to interpret and analyze dreams to gain information about our deepest thoughts and motivations? No we do not. We can interpret our dreams because they are about our issues, but if we already know what our issues are we don't need to waste any time interpreting dreams. Keep in mind that the prefrontal cortex, the part of the brain that controls executive function (judgment, logic, and planning) is deactivated during REM sleep . . . and hence during REM dreams. If we are counting on gaining enlightenment from our dreams we are looking in the wrong place. That would be like deciding to get really drunk before you make some major decisions in you life.

Let's look more at the content of dreams. What do we dream about? Are our dreams just randomly about anything in our lives? No, not really. Dreams are related to the experiences from our most recent waking period.

Joe Griffin did some analysis of dreams and eventually concluded just that (Griffin 2006, 19–25). The fact that we sometimes dredge up past events in our dreams is due to the fact that something in our recent waking experience was directly or indirectly related to that past event. Our mind is attempting to process the current experience by dredging up related experience. Sometimes, without reflection, we might not be aware of what that relationship might be. If our brains did not process, cross-reference, and integrate our recent experience with our past experience then how would we store the memory effectively for later recall? This is how we learn from experience.

This is also why dreams often come across as metaphor. For example, we may have issues going on that we cannot control and if we have enough of these we may start feeling that our lives are out of control. We may end up having a dream about falling. Falling is being out of control, and we dream about falling because of the sensation we are having of being out of control.

Our dreams also tend to be visual in nature. It is difficult to visualize the sensation of being out of control, but we can visualize falling. So the emotion comes across as something visual . . . hence we see ourselves falling. Feeling pressured or not up to a task may come across in our dreams as being chased or walking into a classroom to take a test for which we did not study. Again, these are visual metaphors for what our gut is telling us.

While dreams are mostly visual in nature, like watching through the window while the pizza chef throws dough, the visual cortex is almost completely inactive during dreams. However, areas involved in the analysis of visual scenes and areas involved in visual memory are active (Linden 2007, 214). It is also interesting that even blind people who have lost their sight after about the age of seven or eight continue to dream in mostly visual images (Martin 2002, 176), while individuals who have been blind from birth do not dream in images.

Another interesting fact is that our REM dreams often tend to be negative. Why would that be? The answer is simple. It is the negative stuff in our lives that we tend to need more time and effort processing; hence it is the negative stuff that we tend to dream about because the brain is attempting to process it. Children have more negative stuff to process because they do not have the life experiences to understand loss, emotions, relationships, and so forth. Again, this is why they have more nightmares.

Our brains have also adapted in another interesting way which impacts both our waking world and our dream experience. Our brains attempt to create a coherent, gap-free story from the data they take in (Linden 2007, 225). Our brains try to understand, to make sense of the information they receive. Our brains are not content to perceive information that does not seem to make sense and leave it at that. The brain tries to figure it out, process it, fit it together in some meaningful whole. This is why mystery novels or mysteries on television are so popular, they tap in to the fact that our brains want to figure out how it all fits together . . . to make sense of it . . . to make it coherent.

This same human attribute is what drives us to religious thought (Linden 2007, 225). When the brain is faced with a mystery, with an event or pattern of events it cannot explain, it makes a story from whatever bits and pieces of experience it can dredge up. Hence we have the mystical experience, the miracle, or some sort of divine intervention.

The same thing happens with dreams. The brain is attempting to process experiences into memory, hence it dredges up old memories that might be somehow related in order to file the new memories in a way that best insures the possibility of future retrieval of these memories. As our conscious mind watches this process it attempts to make it into a coherent story. At least it makes it into the best coherent story it can since the prefrontal cortex (logic) is shut down during this phase. Hence our dreams sometimes take on the aura of visions, or prophecies, or mystical and religious experiences, or even nightmares.

There are some very unusual case studies that point out this propensity we have for making sense of mysteries . . . of things we really don't understand. There have been some studies with split brain patients that revealed this. This refers to individuals who had severe seizure activity and surgery was necessary to stop or reduce the seizure activity and give these individuals a somewhat normal life. In these cases the seizures were caused by the flood of information between the two hemispheres of the brain, and the corrective surgery separated the left and right hemispheres of the brain.

A result of this split brain surgery, however, is that now the hemispheres do not and cannot communicate. Hence, if one of these patients saw an object with only one eye, only the hemisphere of the brain that perceived that object could respond to that object. The other hemisphere would have no idea the object was even there. Consequently, if these patients were shown two different pictures, one that could only be seen by the left eye and one that could only be seen by the right eye, the brain could respond to both. However, the brain could not explain both because the locus of control for language is in the left hemisphere (for adults), and the left hemisphere could not explain what the right hemisphere had perceived or reacted to.

This is a very interesting situation. Experimentally some of these patients were shown two pictures, one that could be seen by only the right eye and one only by the left eye (Linden 2007, 227). The right eye (which actually sends information to the left hemisphere and vice versa) was shown a picture of a chicken's foot (claw). The left eye saw a picture of a snowstorm. The patients were then shown other photos (again with each eye) and asked to select pictures that in some way matched or went with the pictures they originally saw. The right eye selected a picture of a chicken, which went with the chicken foot it had seen earlier. The left eye selected a shovel, which could be used to dig out or shovel a driveway after a snowstorm.

Although the hemispheres of the brain could both function and select the appropriate matching items, when the patients were asked why they had selected a chicken and a shovel the responses were interesting. These patients stated that they had selected the chicken because of the chicken foot or claw they had seen, and that they selected the shovel because it could be used to clean out the chicken coop. The left hemisphere, which controls language, had no knowledge of the picture of the snow storm. However, rather than making some comment about not knowing why the shovel was selected, the left hemisphere made some sense of it. It solved the mystery. It made a coherent, believable explanation from the information it had.

In a related experiment (Linden 2007, 229) one of these patients was shown a note but only so the left eye could see it, and hence the information went only to the right hemisphere. The note instructed the patient to go take a walk. As the patient was getting up to do so he was asked where he was going. His left hemisphere, which is the hemisphere that had to respond to the question, had no clue. What the patient said was that he was going to get a drink of water. His left hemisphere was making a plausible attempt to explain his behavior (Linden 2007, 226). The response was never, "I don't know."

Amnesia patients have demonstrated similar behaviors. There are some patients who have brain damage to the extent that they cannot process into memory anything that happened from the previous day. So if you ask one of these patients what they did yesterday they really cannot tell you accurately because they cannot remember. However, when you ask them what they did yesterday they always tell you something. They are not lying. Their brains are attempting to piece together something plausible that they did, and that's what they report. They never say, "I don't know."

This is also, as stated earlier, what happens with our dreams. Our consciousness, without the aid of our prefrontal cortex, views the pieces of data that the brain is processing and attempts to make some rational, coherent story out of it. And sometimes we end up with some pretty wild dreams or nightmares. Some dreams are interesting, and sometimes they are worthy of conversation because they are certainly conversation pieces, but they are not the material from which we should analyze our deepest motivations. A simple explanation of how this works can sometimes help a child understand and better deal with nightmares and bad dreams.

# Chapter 7

# The Impact of
# Stress on Sleep

*The Four Conditions of Stress and
What Happens in the Brain during Stress*

*A small boy once found a butterfly cocoon. He did not know what it was so he took it home. He took it to his father.*

*"Look what I found," said the boy. "What is it?"*

*"Why it is a butterfly cocoon," answered his father. "If you are lucky a butterfly will eventually emerge from this cocoon."*

*"Wow," said the boy, "a butterfly."*

*"Be very careful with it and watch it every day," said the father.*

*"The boy took the cocoon to his room and watched it every day. Before long a small opening appeared. The boy watched the butterfly for several hours as it struggled to get out of the cocoon. Then it seemed to stop struggling. It appeared to be stuck. The boy wanted to help the butterfly so he took a pair of scissors and he cut open the cocoon. The butterfly then emerged easily, but it looked strange to the boy. It had a swollen body and shriveled wings. Over the next several days the butterfly never changed. Its wings never developed and it soon died never having flown.*

*The boy was very disappointed and went to his father to tell him what had happened.*

*"The mistake was in cutting the cocoon open," said the father. "The butterfly needs to struggle to get out of the cocoon. That struggle forces fluid out of its body and into its wings, and that is what allows it to have wings strong enough to fly."*

*It is the same with stress. We cannot take the stress from another, nor can we manage their stress for them. What we can do is help them learn to manage stress*

*better, and we can support them through the process. That is what they need to
make them strong.*

With an understanding of sleep and the importance of sleep, we can now
turn to the issues related to getting better sleep. Better sleep means both
a better quantity of sleep and a better quality of sleep. Dealing with these
issues includes such things as managing stress and stress levels, dealing
with sleep apnea, developing routines, and managing depression.

Stress is a huge factor in whether any of us sleep well or not. The stress
that adolescents have in their lives, how they manage that stress, and how
they think about that stress all play a role in how well they sleep at night.
In the next chapter we will discuss how to manage stress, but first it is
critical to spend some time understanding stress.

When discussing stress it is always good to begin by reminding people
that the brain is a phenomenal organ. Everything we are begins and ends
with that organ between our ears. The thoughts we have are real. They
are measurable to a degree. Every thought we have causes chemicals to be
released in our brains. Every thought we have induces electrical impulses
in the brain. These can be measured.

Our thoughts also cause real physical reactions in our bodies, and those
can be measured. If we think about typical polygraph tests, more com-
monly known as lie detector tests, what do they measure? They do not
measure lies. They measure physiological responses . . . they measure our
stress response. That is because most of us have a stress response when
we lie.

The typical polygraph test measures such things as hand temperature,
heart rate, blood pressure, breathing rate, muscle tension, and perspiration. A stress response causes the hand temperature to decrease. The
hands become cooler because blood flow is being diverted from the ex-
tremities, from the hands and feet, to the major muscle groups for fight
or flight. Our arms and legs need more blood in case we have to run or
fight to protect ourselves, so our hands and feet get less blood during
fight or flight.

Have you ever noticed that your fingers don't seem to function well
when you are under stress and attempting to do something that requires
dexterity? Part of that is the lack of focus due to the stress, but a part of it
is also the decreased blood and oxygen flow to the hands.

A stress response also causes the heart rate to increase. The heart must
pump more blood for the fight-or-flight response. It must pump more
blood so the muscle tissues get the extra oxygen they need to run or
fight.

Blood pressure also increases during a stress response. The heart is pumping more blood and it is pumping it faster . . . again for fight or flight.

A stress response causes the breathing rate to accelerate. The lungs are doing their part to get us more oxygen for fight or flight.

Our muscle tension is higher in a stress response because our muscles are primed for the possible action of fight or flight.

Finally, we perspire more when we have a stress response because our bodies are working a lot harder preparing us for fight or flight.

A relaxation response has just the opposite effect. Our hands become warmer, our heart rate decreases, our blood pressure returns to normal, our breathing rate slows, our muscles relax, and we perspire less. These physiological responses are a dead giveaway as to the truth or lies that we are telling . . . at least for most people. People can be trained to have some control over their physiological responses, and those few among us who are true sociopaths and have no remorse over what they say or what they do may not have the same physiological responses. For most of us, however, a lie detector test demonstrates the stress we are experiencing.

It is interesting to note that sometimes when we talk to a child, or anyone really, the physical reactions we see in the body do not match the words coming out of the mouth. They say something like, "No, I am not angry!" but they say it emphatically with their arms defiantly crossed over their chest, their jaw set, their teeth clenched, and their eyes looking daggers through you. In those cases it is pretty clear that, in fact, they are angry.

In those instances it is important to understand that the truth always lies in the physical responses we are seeing rather than in the words coming out of someone's mouth. It is fairly easy for most of us to lie with our words, but it is very difficult to mask our physical or our physiological responses. We certainly can misinterpret someone's physical response, but the truth is always in the physical response rather than with the words. That is why lie detector tests work for most people.

So what causes this stress response? What are the conditions that evoke stress in us? There are four conditions that create stress (Plaford 2006, 75). These are novelty, unpredictability, lack of control, and threat to ego. Every stress that we face, every stress that our children or our loved ones face, every stress that our co-workers or colleagues face, every stress that our employees or our supervisors face fall under one or more of these four conditions. If we understand these conditions, and which one or which ones of these are creating a specific stress, then we can more accurately and effectively help to find interventions to address the specific stressor.

Let's look at these four conditions more closely. What is novelty? Novelty refers to a new situation, something we are not accustomed to. Change is an example of novelty. Change causes stress in us even if it is change that we want, that we look forward to. Getting married, even though it is a choice that we are willingly making and even anticipating, causes a certain amount of stress. Changing schools causes stress, whether it is because of moving to a new city or moving from elementary school to middle school. Often, although not always, adults have choices regarding the changes in their lives. In many respects children have no choice regarding such changes.

Additionally, some people will resist change at all cost. They will dig in their heels and try desperately to cling to the old routine and fight tooth and nail over doing something in a different manner. Know anyone like that?

A favorite book is one by Dr. Spencer Johnson entitled, *Who Moved My Cheese?* (1998). It is about four characters, two mice and two human-like characters, who live in a maze. How they respond when the cheese is moved, when change occurs, is the subject of the book. A favorite line in that book is a question that is repeated several times throughout the book. The question is, "What would I do if I weren't afraid?" That is a very powerful question. "What would I do if I weren't afraid?" It is powerful because the fear that comes from stress can disrupt how we function. It can disrupt our ability to function. So, "What would I do if I weren't afraid to function?" "How would I handle this situation then?"

That is such a powerful question that it can be used on the golf course. In playing competitive golf there are often times when stress comes into play. There are times when it is easy to look at the obstacles rather than the goal. There are times it is easy to hit a shot thinking about what we don't want to happen rather than thinking about what we do want to happen. "I don't want to hit the ball in the lake." That fearful thinking most often results in poor shot making. So asking yourself what you would do if you weren't afraid to hit this shot refocuses your thinking on the goal, and it allows you to hit better shots. The point is that novelty and change are huge stressors, and that the resulting fear and anxiety that come with them often disrupt our ability to function as we would like.

Another condition that creates stress is that of unpredictability. Unpredictability means that something is about to happen but we don't know what . . . we cannot predict it. The expectation is stressful. In reality we often expect more severe results than what actually happens. This is called impact bias (Gilbert, 2002).

This unpredictability factor is a staple of horror movies. The hero or heroine is about to open the door, but what is on the other side of the door? Or they are about to put their hand in the water or even jump into the water, but what is in the water just under the surface? Or we see the corn stalks moving . . . what is in the corn field? The music will usually build at this time warning us that something is about to happen. The moviemaker is creating stress and anxiety in the viewer by using unpredictability because unpredictability is a huge stressor.

A third condition that creates stress is lack of control. This is when something is about to happen and we cannot control it, or we are afraid we cannot control it. This feeling of lack of control is another staple of horror movies. In fact the most horrifying movies they have ever made are the ones where the demon, being, creature, microbe, or whatever actually enters the person's body and takes over. That is really loss of control, and that is more terrifying than death itself. If we just have death in a movie it is an adventure film, or possibly a bloodbath adventure film. It is the lack of control and the unpredictability that turns the movie into horror.

Movie directors will also use the lack of control factor by putting the hero or the heroine in a situation where they have no control. For example, they will put the heroine in a coffin in the ground. There is nothing she can do . . . she has absolutely no control . . . if she is going to be saved someone else will have to save her.

Horror movie producers will often use lack of control and unpredictability together to get an even more terrifying response. They will chain the heroine to the wall (lack of control), and then we hear something crawling down the hallway toward her (unpredictability). At those moments when our heart is in our throat, so to speak, they have successfully elevated our stress level.

Do you know anyone you would term a control freak? That is another instance where we see the lack of control factor. The control freak has learned that when they control everything their own stress level is lower, and when they are not in control their stress level elevates. So attempting to control everything is an attempt to manage their own stress or possibly avoid stress. It may create more stress in you dealing with that individual, but it is all about stress.

What about conditions such as claustrophobia? What is claustrophobia all about? Claustrophobia is when we have a fear of being in an enclosed or narrow space. What happens if we are in a close or tight space? We cannot move around. If it is tight enough we cannot move at all . . . like being wedged between the walls in a cave. Not being able to move is all about a lack of control. This is a control issue. The fear of heights or the fear of falling is the same. Those are fears about falling out of control. When events in our lives really feel out of control, what is it we often dream about? Falling! We have nightmares about falling. These are all issues of control or lack of control. Lack of control is a huge, huge stressor.

The final condition that causes stress is threat to ego. This can refer to an actual threat to our life or well-being like being shot at in a war zone, being mugged in an alley, or being in an automobile accident when we thought we were going to die. Threat to ego also refers to symbolic threats. This would include being put down, overlooked, unappreciated, disrespected or "dissed" as youth say, losing face, or losing esteem.

An example of threat to ego often comes with public speaking. Many people are terrified of public speaking. It is a huge fear. I have heard friends state that they would rather jump out of an airplane than have to speak in front of a crowd. If they were actually given that choice they probably would not choose jumping out of the airplane, but the fact is they are placing public speaking at that level of fear in their eyes. Jumping out of an airplane is dangerous, while public speaking is not dangerous. However, public speaking is a threat to ego. There is the threat that we will look foolish, that we will forget what we were going to say and loose esteem, that we will not be as respected if we somehow mess up.

We also see the threat to ego factor in sports. In amateur golf tournaments, for example, why do some golfers choke? It is the fear of looking bad, or loosing esteem, or making a fool out of themselves that causes them to do exactly what they are afraid of doing. They choke because of the threat to ego. Threat to ego is a major stressor.

These four conditions are the conditions that create stress. Understanding these conditions and understanding which of these conditions is generating a specific stress in us can help us understand how to intervene in our stress, or in the stress of our loved ones.

One situation where stress can often be observed is on the first day of school. Freshmen entering their high school experience will often be stressed the first few days. Sixth or seventh grade students entering their first middle school experience will be stressed. Kindergarten or first grade students will often feel stress that first day of school.

At the elementary level we often see especially high levels of stress in those children who have never been in a school experience before. While many children have had preschool experiences of some kind, some have not. Those who have not, those for whom this first day of school is really their first day of school ever, will sometimes have a meltdown. What we see is a hallway tantrum. The child is clinging to the parent, crying, screaming, and/or pleading not to be left. This is typically because of the novelty and/or unpredictability of the experience. The parent is trying to pry the child's fingers away from her dress but may also be fighting back tears because of the trauma her child is experiencing. The teacher is telling the parent to just leave, let us handle it. The parent does not know what to do.

These scenes could be avoided in most cases by taking the child to the open house that was held at the school for new students, usually scheduled a few days prior to the first day. At this open house the child would meet the teacher, walk around the room, sit in a chair at a desk, and generally see what is going on. This addresses the novelty and unpredictability factors, and is generally enough to alleviate the child's stress or at least the high level of stress that otherwise results in the hallway tantrum.

A similar situation in which we see stress is when the child is picked up by the school bus the very first time. Again, it is the novelty and unpredictability that causes some children to be reluctant or even refuse to get on the school bus. Some schools have addressed this by having a school bus at the open house and encouraging parents of kindergarten and first grade students to take their children on the bus, walk around, sit in a seat. This addresses the novelty and unpredictability related to the bus, and decreases the child's stress level.

Understanding the condition or conditions that cause stress in our lives, the lives of our children and loved ones, or the lives of those we work with as either clients or co-workers can help us know how to plan interventions that are meaningful to reduce stress. If we address the condition or conditions that are causing the stress, we will be more effective than if we just throw out stress reduction generalities.

What happens in the brain when we experience stress? One of the first things that happens is that cortisol levels increase. Cortisol is a neurotransmitter that begins to ready the body for fight or flight (Plaford 2006, 75). It is often called the "stress hormone" because of its involvement in our response to stress. Stress elevates cortisol levels and, interestingly, so does sleep deprivation. Cortisol interacts with other agents in the body like adrenalin, epinephrine, and norepinephrine to increase blood pressure, inhibit the immune system response and inflammation, and break down lipids and proteins to create a higher glucose level in the blood system. All of these act to ready our bodies for fight or flight.

Along with higher levels of cortisol the brain decreases the level of serotonin. Serotonin is a neurotransmitter that calms or soothes us, and it suppresses anger and aggression. One of the functions of antidepressant medications, like Prozac, is to increase the level of serotonin in the brain to soothe depression. Prozac does not actually increase serotonin levels, but rather it inhibits the re-uptake of serotonin thereby keeping serotonin in the synapses longer.

The combination of increased cortisol and decreased serotonin levels in the body primes us for the fight-or-flight response, sometimes called the acute stress response. The fight-or-flight response is a normal, natural response that we have when we perceive danger. The amygdala, part of the limbic system, is a key player in our recognition of fear and therefore in the activation of the fight-or-flight response. When we take a walk in the woods, for example, and we are suddenly startled because we almost stepped on a snake, our response is to jump back. We are breathing harder at this point, and our heart rate has accelerated pumping more blood.

Then the neocortex kicks in and we notice that the snake has not moved. Eventually we realize that it isn't a snake at all but rather a stick. Our breathing begins to return to normal and our heart rate begins to slow. The point is, however, that the limbic system does not wait for the neocortex to figure out all the clues before it responds. If the amygdala perceives danger it will kick in the fight-or-flight response and literally take over our functioning.

If you have ever tried to talk to someone who was really terrified you know what I mean. You can be right in the person's face screaming for them to listen to you, but they can't. Their eyes are darting everywhere, watching for danger cues, and they are prepared to fight or run. It is incredibly difficult for them to focus on language, on what you are saying, at that point.

Despite the problems it sometimes causes us, the fight-or-flight response is a normal and natural response. It is designed to save our lives. We need this response. There have been studies where researchers have surgically removed the amygdala from rats. These rats became fearless rats. They would become hungry, they would see food, and they would also see a cat. They showed no fear of the cat, however, and would go after the food. These rats were killed very quickly. They did not live long because when they needed to be afraid, when they needed the fight-or-flight response, it was not initiated.

We need the fight-or-flight response. The problem is that it sometimes kicks in when we wish it would not. It can cause a disruption to our functioning, and it can have some very negative long-term effects. It can be disrupting when we need to make a speech, for example. Our stress level rises because of our perceived threat to ego, and the fight-or-flight response kicks in and we have trouble focusing on what we want to say.

Long term there are much more significant problems. High levels of cortisol in the brain and body for extended periods can suppress thyroid functioning, decrease bone density, decrease muscle tone and muscle density and thereby increase abdominal fat which is related to stroke and heart attack. It can also lower our immune response, it can cause higher blood pressure, it can cause hyperglycemia, which can be a precursor to diabetes, and it can damage the hippocampus which impairs cognitive function. These are all fairly serious side effects of prolonged, high levels of cortisol. The one that is possibly the most serious is that it can damage the hippocampus.

There have been some interesting studies done with post-traumatic stress disorder patients, and one of the factors that we see is a damaged, decreased, shrunken hippocampus. A lot of soldiers with PTSD have been studied because being in a war zone, being shot at regularly, generates high levels of stress over a long period. Consequently, the hippocampus is shrunken, depleted, or damaged.

Sonjia Lupine (2004), a researcher at McGill University, has recently studied PTSD patients and their siblings. Siblings were included in the study because it has been noticed that some siblings of PTSD patients also have a damaged, depleted hippocampus. These are not PTSD patients themselves, but merely siblings of PTSD patients. Why would they have a damaged hippocampus?

When they took social histories of the PTSD patients and these siblings they found that as children these individuals grew up in homes where they faced high levels of stress. Childhood stress, with the resulting high levels of cortisol, can be a precursor to post-traumatic stress disorder. Not only does intense exposure to cortisol damage the hippocampus, but in children such intense exposure to cortisol may keep the hippocampus from developing to its full potential. This is because the brain is still developing in children.

Regardless of how it impacts the hippocampus, we know it does. We also know that childhood stress can set people up for post-traumatic stress disorder if they face high levels of stress or trauma later on in life.

So what causes stress in children? There are a number of things that can do this. Growing up in poverty is one huge stressor. We can see this if we look at the conditions that cause stress in relation to poverty. First of all, children who grow up in poverty often face a great deal of novelty in their lives. One week it may be mom and the kids living in an apartment, and the next week mom gets a new boyfriend and moves in with him. Now there is a new family structure, another new authority figure, a new neighborhood; his children from a different marriage may be there on occasion; there will be a new school, a new teacher, new classmates, and so forth.

Several months later mom breaks up with this boyfriend and moves in with grandma. Now there is another new family structure, another new set of rules, another new neighborhood, another new school, another new teacher, etc. Some children in poverty move like this three or four times a year . . . every year. That is a lot of change and a lot of stress.

Growing up in poverty also creates a great deal of unpredictability. With all the moving around that comes with poverty a child learns to expect the unexpected. Since they keep moving, is it worth the effort to try to make friends at this school or with this teacher? Is it worth the effort to try, once again, to get caught up with the class on what they are learning? How long will they be in this class in this school? That is stressful.

They also face the unpredictability of whether there will be food when they get home at night. Will mom even be there? If she is there will she be drunk or high on drugs again? If she is drunk will she be passed out? If she isn't passed out, will she be happy, cuddly drunk or will she be mean drunk where she hurts us? Will the police show up again like they did last week? All of this unpredictability creates stress for the child.

Additionally, children growing up in poverty have very little control over the situation, and they begin to internalize that sense of a lack of control. There has been research where children in poverty and children not in poverty were asked questions about the world and what is possible in the world. Children who are not living in poverty believe that things are possible, and they believe that they can be anything or do anything when they grow up. Children who are living in poverty don't answer the same way. They start to believe that things are not possible and that they cannot be anything or do anything in life.

They also start to believe more in luck, fate, and chance. If life is all about luck, fate, and chance, then why try in the first place? This sense of no control results in a lack of effort to make changes. If we don't believe that we can make changes, that we can influence our futures, then why make the effort?

Finally, growing up in poverty is a threat to ego. Children growing up in poverty don't typically do as well in school as children who do not live in poverty. This is not because they are not as smart or not as capable, but rather because all the moving around has created huge gaps in their education. They have missed things educationally that they need in order to make sense of what they are currently studying. They have often not been read to at home and language is not used by the parent as a tool to promote literacy. They also have typically not been asked the same kind of questions at home like, "What did you do in school today? Did you get your homework done? Can I see your homework? Do you understand this?" These children have also been more focused on survival than on getting their schoolwork done.

The upshot is that they don't do as well in school, but they interpret that as not being as smart or as capable as their peers. That is a threat to ego, which results in less effort, falling further behind, doing even worse academically, and feeling even more incapable of competing in life.

Another situation that causes stress in childhood is being regularly abused or neglected. Every time a child is abused it is novel, it is different. It is always unpredictable . . . they never know when it will happen again. They feel they have no control over it. And it is a threat to ego . . . they must be horrible children to keep making daddy so angry that he hurts them. How many children in our society face abuse and neglect on a regular basis? This is a huge stressor in their lives.

Growing up with domestic violence is another childhood stressor. Seeing mom beaten up by dad on a regular basis is stressful. It may be dad or it may be a string of live-in boyfriends, but the result is incredibly stressful for the child who witnesses it.

Finally, what about bullying? Being bullied on a regular basis puts a child under tremendous stress. Every time a child is bullied it is novel. It is always unpredictable, which is why children who are bullied tend to miss school. They avoid school because they never know when they will be bullied again. They feel a definite lack of control. They think that the bully has all the control. Victims are often reluctant to tell the teacher or other authorities at school because they don't think those people can stop the bully. They sense that all the power is with the bully. Being bullied is also a threat to ego and it is sometimes a double-whammy threat to ego. The bullied child will wonder why me, what is wrong with me, why don't I fit in? They will also debase themselves for not having the courage, the backbone, the intelligence to stand up for themselves.

There are other stressors that children may grow up with. The death of a parent and the subsequent financial and emotional instability that causes for the family is a stressor. A parent who has poor health but lingers on the verge of death for years is another example. The point is, high levels of childhood stress can damage the hippocampus and therefore put a child at risk of not being able to manage stress well the rest of their life.

One other aspect regarding stress must be mentioned before we move on. That relates to stress levels. There are times in our lives when we experience no stress, mild stress, moderate stress, and high stress. Levels of stress impact us differently. Having no stress, or being in a comfort zone, is like being in a hammock on the beach. There is a gentle breeze, the sound of the surf, the hammock is gently swaying, there is a cool drink at our side, everything is perfect. We are experiencing no stress and we are not motivated to move or make any changes.

When we experience mild stress we start to think about what we need to do to make the situation better. There may be a little sand in the hammock, or the sun may have moved around the corner of the shade tree and is now in our face. So we get up, shake out the hammock or move the hammock further into the shade. We do something to address the minor stress.

When we face minor stress at work we begin to think about what we can do to improve the situation. Do we need to have a discussion with that colleague, do we need to buy them a cup of coffee, do we need to just avoid them for awhile, or possibly talk to the supervisor? How can we make things better?

At school, teachers create mild stress in students all the time by announcing that there will be a test on Friday. Most students will do something to address the stress, and we hope they will do more than pray. They may pray, but what they will also do is study. If they know the material it will reduce their stress. Basically they study to reduce their stress level.

When we move into a high level of stress we are moving into fight or flight. In high stress we are not looking at how to improve the situation. Rather we are looking at how we can get away from or out of the situation. If we have a job that constantly puts us under high levels of stress what do we do? We start looking for another job. Most of us won't stay in a highly stressful job for long unless there are rewards sufficient enough that we deem worth the stress. The student who is put under high stress by the announcement of the test on Friday won't show up on Friday.

The point is that while mild stress may be motivational, high stress often results in running away from the stress. Consequently, individuals who face high levels of stress during childhood can very easily get into a pattern of running away, of avoiding stress and/or situations that cause stress. They don't learn to face problems, to solve problems, they learn to run from problems. They get into a pattern of running away. We see this in individuals in a relationship who run away when the relationship hits a rough spot. They don't stick around to work things out . . . they are out of there. How many one-parent families do we have because of that very reason?

Stress is an ever present factor in our lives and in the lives of our children and students, and it is a factor that we must teach our children to manage rather than run away from. The stress that a child or adolescent faces certainly can have a major impact on that child's education. It impacts their health and it certainly impacts their sleep. Their sleep can be impacted in several ways. Moderate levels of stress often lead to increased amounts of REM sleep, while high levels of stress tend to reduce the total amount of sleep achieved (Siegel 2001, 1058–63). Since stress does so significantly impact both the quantity and the quality of sleep, how do we manage stress and how do we teach our children to do so?

# Chapter 8

# Managing Stress

## Understanding Emotions and Brain Functioning

*Thomas Alva Edison invented the practical, usable version of the lightbulb as we know it. But Thomas Edison tested over three thousand filaments before he developed one that was both durable and practical. Some people would say that he failed three thousand times before he was successful, but that isn't what Thomas Edison said. He said, "Results . . . I have gotten results! If I find 10,000 ways something won't work, I haven't failed . . . because every wrong attempt discarded is often a step forward."*

*The way we look at things, our mindset, our habitual ways of thinking, our habitual thought patterns are critical in how we interpret life. And how we interpret life determines our ultimate success or failure in life.*

Managing stress is important, but managing stress is difficult for most people, and it can't be done with a recipe book. We cannot just provide a few tips to use and these will allow children to be victorious over stress. It is important to have strategies; these are useful, but it is also helpful to have a little better understanding about some other factors that are involved in stress. For example, it is valuable to have some understanding of how the brain functions.

Understanding the limbic system and how it functions is one piece of the puzzle. The limbic system is the emotional center of the brain. It is also beneficial to understand a little of how the brain hemispheres work together because the locus of control of brain functioning can and does shift between these hemispheres. The knowledge that the locus of control does shift means that we can learn to shift it at our will, which means we can teach children and adolescents to do the same. If they can have some control over this shift, they can learn how to calm themselves at will.

It is also advantageous to have some understanding of emotional intelligence. Part of emotional intelligence is being able to manage emotions and delay gratification. The higher level of emotional intelligence children have, the better capability they have of managing their emotions and controlling the stress in their lives.

Another factor that is critical to understand is that of habitual thought patterns or mindset. The way children habitually think about things, the mindset they have when they interpret issues, determines whether they have stress and the level of that stress when facing issues.

We will discuss each of these topics in turn. Let's begin by discussing the functioning of the limbic system. One of the functions, which was discussed in the previous chapter, is that it perceives danger cues and kicks in the fight-or-flight response. That is an important function. Another function of the limbic system, which was mentioned in chapter 4, has to do with memory. The limbic system plays a key role in processing experiences into long term memory (Linden 2007, 16). It also stores memory short term in the hippocampus. The limbic system is especially important in processing emotional memories.

If we live through some really horrifying experience, the emotions we felt during that experience are stored in the hippocampus exactly as we experienced them. For example, we are in a car wreck and the car is turning somersaults. We think we are about to die. All the horror, all the terror, all the anxiety, all the lack of control is stored exactly as we felt it. But somehow we don't die, we walk away. Our brain must then process that emotional experience to store it in memory so that we learn from it and hopefully don't make the same driving mistake again.

The brain processes such experience, in this case the accident, through REM sleep. If REM sleep is shut down, however, we don't process those emotions. How is REM sleep shut down? There are several possibilities. First, our own biochemical reactions can shut down REM sleep if the event was traumatic enough. Secondly, we sometimes self-medicate when we have traumatic experiences. We use alcohol or street drugs or other medications from the medicine cabinet and we dull our senses to try to obliterate the experience. Or possibly we had an injury during the accident, our arm was smashed or mangled and we are on strong pain medications. Any of those things can shut down REM sleep.

When REM sleep is shut down, and we don't process the emotional reactions we had during such an accident, what then happens? We end up with a post-traumatic stress response. What happens with post-traumatic stress disorder is that the emotions experienced during an event keep coming back with all the horror, all the terror, all the anxiety, all the lack of control that we felt during the original experience. The emotions have not been processed and, hence, we keep reliving them. We don't have a processed memory of them . . . we are reliving them exactly as we experienced them. The role our limbic system plays in emotional memory is a key role in our lives, because when that process is disrupted we can have serious problems.

Another role the limbic system plays, specifically the amygdala, is to color our experiences emotionally (Amen 1998, 39). By doing that it gives us preferences, and our preferences are key in decision making. Have you ever gone to a movie that a friend suggested was really good, and you hated it? Or have you ever recommended a movie that you loved, and your friend hated it? Sometimes we are quite surprised that others don't have the same reaction to a movie that we had. The reason they don't is that we are all processing that movie through our own lenses . . . our own preferences . . . and that is also based on our past preferences.

Have you ever read a movie review and the critics are all giving the movie a big thumbs up and piling on the accolades, but you don't like the stars in the movie and, therefore, you decide not to see it? Or just the reverse, the critics pan a movie but you like the stars so you see it anyway? We are using our preferences to make decisions, and they truly help us make decisions.

Likewise, we all have preferences when it comes to ice cream flavors. If you went to an ice cream parlor with thirty-some flavors and you had no preferences, how would you ever make a decision? There have been case studies with individuals who had damage to their amygdalae, and one of the consequences was that they had a terrible time making even simple decisions. Our preferences are key in helping us make decisions.

Our emotions are also crucial in our decision making. For example, two high school boys get into a fight at school and are sent to the principal's office. There the principal or assistant principal starts talking to the boys and finds out that the fight was over a girl. She was dating one of these boys, but she dumped him and is now going out with the other. There are feelings of jealousy, rage, resentment, loss, anger, loss of esteem, and on and on.

The decisions that resulted in the fight were made out of emotions. Probably 99 percent, or more, of the discipline problems that end up in the office in high schools are the result of decisions made out of emotions. If we could teach our children how to manage their emotions better we would have a huge impact in decreasing school discipline issues.

Let's bring this closer to home. What are you doing next Friday night? We sometimes have responsibilities, especially if we are parents, and sometimes we delay gratification because we have a project to complete.

However, when we have free time, and for many of us Friday nights are considered our free time, we most often fill that time with things we enjoy. That is when we can forget about work and do what we want.

That is exactly what we typically do. We forget our problems and do something that makes us feel good. That may be different at times depending on our energy level and our state of mind, but we do fun things . . . enjoyable things.

Sometimes that may be going out for a nice dinner. Sometimes it might mean staying at home by the fire with a good book. Sometimes it might mean going out with friends to party. The point is, we do what we think will make us happy. We make that decision based on emotion . . . happiness. You can bet that children and adolescents make decisions about what they are going to do based on what they think will make them feel good. It is emotion that drives much of their decision making.

There was an interesting study done at Princeton University (Restak 2003, 113–14). Subjects were given the following scenario. You, the subject, are in charge of a train station. You work in a work station far above and overlooking the tracks below. You see a train coming very quickly down the tracks to your right. It will soon round a curve and be right below you. You look below and see five individuals on the tracks. These people should not be there, but there they are. They are in a location where the walls are very high on both sides of the track, and they could not possibly get off the track when the train comes into view. These people will die shortly unless you do something.

So what are your options? You can push a button and switch the train to another track, but when you look at that track there is one individual on it. Again, he should not be there, but there he is. He also would not be able to get off the track when he sees the train. So you must make a choice. What do you do?

Most of the subjects decided they would push the button and switch the train to the track with only one person on it. When asked why they made that choice they rationalized that they, reluctantly, had to. Saving five for one was the right thing to do. The math made sense, five for one . . . one for five. They had no other choice.

Then the scenario was changed. They were given the following, similar scenario. You are not in charge of the station but you work there. You are on a platform overlooking the tracks and you see the same train coming. You also see these same five people on the tracks. If you don't do something these five individuals will soon die. You also know something about trains. If a train hits something it will automatically come to a screeching halt.

In this scenario there is another individual on the platform with you. You don't know this person, but he is hanging way out over the platform watching the scene that is about to take place below. If you push him he will fall on the track. The train will hit him and he will die, but the train will stop and the five individuals on the track will be saved. Again, what do you do?

The subjects, in this scenario, could not push the other individual off the platform to save the five individuals down below. They chose to let the five die. Here is the interesting point. . .the math is the same. It is still five for one or one for five, but the subjects could not make that decision.

We make many decisions in our lives, and many of those we rationalize with logic—it makes sense to do it—but that does not always mean the decision was based on logic. Emotions play a huge part in the decisions that we make. They are a powerful part of the process, and we must consider that and accept the role they play in our lives. We tend to dismiss our emotions, and if we show them at all, especially for men, we feel we are being weak. Not true. If we acknowledge the role emotions play we could in fact make sounder decisions. We need to teach this to our children.

Let's take it one step further. What about motivation? What motivates us to accomplish something? What makes the star basketball player the star? Is it merely talent? Certainly there has to be some athletic ability, but the star player becomes the star player by practicing harder and longer than anyone else. It is emotion that drives them to practice. It is the love of the game. It is the love of the ball going through the hoop, or the love of the movement, or the love of the competition, or the love of the crowd noise or the accolades they receive from playing the game. It is the love, the passion that they have for playing and winning at this sport that causes them to put in the hours that it takes to be the best.

Fear will also motivate us, but the motivation from fear typically wanes once the fear stimulus is gone. Some coaches, especially little league coaches, don't get this at all. They try to motivate through fear and intimidation because those coaches don't know how to use and channel passion.

Besides passion and fear, we will also at times be motivated to do things or try things that we like or think we might like. Or we will do things to be with people we like. But when we have to make choices about what we stick to, it is passion or love of something that drives us. All the major accomplishments in the world were achieved out of passion . . . out of love, or sometimes fear. By accomplishments I don't mean discoveries because those can be accidental or unplanned, but I mean accomplishments that individuals had to stick to, had to devote time and energy to, had to make sacrifices to attain. Those accomplishments were all achieved because of passion . . . because of a fire deep inside us . . . because of love . . . because of emotion.

It is emotion that drives motivation. If we can motivate a child to learn, he will learn. On a side note, our government made one of the grandest mistakes of all time with its No Child Left Behind policies. The concept is good . . . no child should be left behind. It is the manner in which the government has tried to achieve No Child Left Behind that is problematic. The focus is on test scores. You cannot achieve this concept with test scores. You get children to learn, and more importantly to want to learn, through motivation. But motivation is based on emotion. We have to build emotional intelligence in our children in order to motivate them. They must be able to recognize emotions, manage emotions, and delay gratification to truly achieve. We will never get that by focusing on test scores. We will get higher test scores by focusing on emotions.

There was a very interesting study done a number of years ago by Walter Mischel of Stanford University (Goleman 1994, 81–83). His study began with four-year-old children. He began by giving each of them an IQ test. After that he spent some time talking with each child individually.

After a short while he stated that he had to leave, but that he would return to finish their conversation. He asked the child to wait for him and he gave each child a marshmallow as a token of appreciation for their participation and for talking with him. This was their marshmallow. They could eat it at any time. However, if they waited until he returned to eat it, they would then receive a second marshmallow. They did not have to wait, but the only way to get a second marshmallow was to wait. It was their decision.

Then he left and watched the children through a two-way mirror. Some of the children ate the marshmallow and some waited and earned the second marshmallow. Those who ate the marshmallow tended to eat it soon after he left. Those who waited and earned the second marshmallow tried all sorts of strategies to not eat the marshmallow. You can almost picture some of these kids and their strategies. They would talk to themselves, talk to the marshmallow, sing to themselves, sing to the marshmallow, stare at the marshmallow, stare at the wall trying not to look at the marshmallow, put their head down to try to nap, and so forth. The strategies worked because some of these children did earn the second marshmallow.

Mischel came back to these kids twelve years later, they were now sixteen-year-old high school students. He looked at how they were doing both academically and socially. Academically the students who had earned the second marshmallow had better grades. Socially they were more dependable, more trustworthy, they stuck to tasks better and did not give up when things were hard.

He came back to these students again two years later. They were now eighteen and taking their SAT exams for college entry. Those students who had earned the second marshmallow scored an average of 210 points higher on their total SAT scores than did the other students. Earning the second marshmallow was more than twice as effective at predicting higher SAT scores than were their IQ scores.

We tend to focus on the wrong things. Emotional intelligence is a far better predictor of success in life than is cognitive intelligence. Yet we still focus on test scores rather than on building emotional intelligence. If we took a saner approach we could focus on building emotional intelligence and hence motivate children, and motivated children will learn. In fact, once you motivate a child, you cannot keep that child from learning.

Understanding our emotions and the limbic system, which is the emotional center of our brain, is important in understanding how we can manage stress. Understanding a little about the right and left hemispheres of the brain is also critical. Dr. Elkonan Goldberg, on the neurology faculty at New York University Medical School, has written a book called *The Executive Brain* (2001). In this book he discusses the locus of control of brain functioning.

We used to think that the locus of control for specific functions of the brain was set in the different hemispheres of the brain. For example, we thought that the locus of control for language was in the left hemisphere and the locus of control for musical ability was in the right hemisphere. When we looked at adults who had strokes it seemed to verify that thinking, because a stroke in the left hemisphere certainly impacted language.

More recently we began to notice strokes in children. Not as many children have strokes as adults, but when a child does have a stroke what was noted is that it was a stroke in the right hemisphere that impacted language. . .not the left. It was totally the reverse from what happens with adults. That caused some researchers to take a step back and realize they did not understand this as well as they thought they had.

This resulted in some interesting studies with children, and a very important concept about how the brain functions was discovered. What was learned is that the locus of control for certain functions will shift. Our brains will shift the locus of control for specific functions, and the basis for that shift is determined by what becomes routine for us. In other words, new or novel experiences will be processed in the right hemisphere, but routine experiences will be processed in the left hemisphere. Whatever functions we perform enough for them to become routine will be shifted to the left hemisphere of the brain.

This makes sense for language. For adults language is processed in the left hemisphere as we always thought. We may learn a new word here and there, but the way we use language is routine, except when we begin to learn a foreign language. If we start to learn Italian, for example, we will process that in the right hemisphere until and/or unless we begin to become proficient in speaking Italian. At that point it would shift to the left hemisphere.

For a child, however, language is novel. Young children have no language. Then they start to learn words like, "Mama" or "Dada." Then they learn to put a few words together, "Me drink." Eventually they are speaking in short sentences and finally longer sentences. At some point the use of language becomes routine enough that the locus of control for language will shift to the left hemisphere of the brain.

That brings up some very interesting questions. For example, we know that some children stutter developmentally, but some children who stutter simply seem to outgrow the stuttering. Why does that happen? Is it that whatever is causing the stuttering is a part of the right hemisphere functioning, and that the "outgrowing" of the stuttering is really that the locus of control has shifted to the left hemisphere? That is not known for sure, but it does bring up some interesting possibilities. Because the locus of control will shift to the left hemisphere for routine experiences, can we shift the locus of control at will from the right hemisphere (problem solving mode) or from the limbic system (stress mode) to the left hemisphere by doing routine things? In fact, we can and we do it all the time.

We can readily see this shift when we examine sports. Golf is a wonderful example, especially amateur golf. If we look at amateur tournaments, city championships, or club championships that are flighted, we regularly see people who choke. We can see it in professional golfers too, but not to the extent that we see it in amateur golf. That isn't merely because of the talent, there is more to it. In amateur matches we often see individuals who can play golf at a certain level but who suddenly can't seem to hit the ball correctly. They make one mistake after another. Sometimes in a match we see both contestants doing this . . . seemingly trying to give the match to each other. They become frustrated and it is frustrating to watch.

What do sports psychologists tell us to do when competing in golf? They have for years told us to get into a routine before we hit the ball. Certainly we must decide how far we are from the green and decide on the proper club to hit, but after that we have to let routine take over. We need to take the same deep breath, we need to have the same swing thoughts, we need to take exactly the same practice swing, we need to step up to the ball exactly the same way, we need to take exactly the same waggle before the shot. If we do these things we hit the ball better.

This works, and we know it works, but why does it work? It works because what we are doing is shifting the locus of control to the left hemisphere. We are shifting it out of the limbic system where stress, specifically threat to ego, is taking over. By shifting the locus to the left hemisphere, we get our stress out of the way and let our bodies do what we have taught them to do.

The same is true of basketball. Basketball is a fast-paced, emotional game. The players run up and down the court at full speed until someone is fouled. Then everything stops and one player steps to the free throw line to shoot free throws. What do all good free throw shooters have in common? They all have a routine they use to shoot free throws.

If a basketball coach is interested in improving his team's free throw shooting, the first thing he should do with his players is to make sure they all have a free throw routine. Those players who tend to choke the worst during game competition should have longer routines. Then during the actual game they should not think about the free throw, but merely go through their routines and let the free throw shot take care of itself. They would make more free throws by doing that because they would be shifting the locus of control, by utilizing routine, to the left hemisphere.

In 2004, the Summer Olympics was held in Athens, Greece. Two divers from the United States team made the finals in the women's platform diving competition. During the competition one of the divers, Laura Wilkinson, who had won the gold medal in the 2000 Olympics, was asked how she dove.

She responded that she dove "brain dead." The interviewer then asked her what she meant by "brain dead?" She replied that she knew these dives very well. She had practiced them repeatedly. If she thought about the dives too much during the competition (right hemisphere), she would mess up. And if she thought about the dives she would also become stressed (limbic system), and then she would really mess up. What she had to do was simply go through her routines (left hemisphere), and let her body do what she had taught it to do. She was not using the terms right hemisphere, left hemisphere, or limbic system . . . but that is exactly what she was talking about and exactly what she was doing.

Handling grief and trauma is another example of how the locus of control can be shifted. Grief and trauma are not the same thing. Grief is a natural response to loss. It is a healing response. We must go through grief to heal. If we do not grieve we do not heal. If we stuff a loss, then the next loss that comes along brings this loss back again full force, and we are then dealing with both. Trauma, on the other hand, is being stuck in the loss experience. Trauma is not being able to move into grief.

Cheri Lovre (2004), a well-known crisis intervention specialist, once gave the following example during a speaking engagement. She spoke of a woman who was stuck in trauma. The trauma was that her daughter had been shot to death by a gunman. All of the woman's thoughts were about the fact that her daughter was now dead. She would never graduate from high school. She would never go to the prom. She would never get the opportunity to go to college. Her life was ended prematurely by this gunman.

This woman tried to get counseling for herself, but the counselor continued to ask her what she felt about her daughter's death. All she could think about was her daughter's death, but her feelings were multiple and were difficult to put into words. She stopped going to counseling very quickly.

She was also having nightmares, and the nightmares were always the same. In her dreams she would see her daughter standing there. She would see the gunman standing there. She would see the gunman pointing the gun at her daughter. She would see the gunman start to pull the trigger. That is where she would wake up, with her heart pounding and in a panic.

Someone who knew how the brain functions asked her to tell the story of her daughter's life. She could do that. She could put that into words. While she could not talk about her feelings as such regarding her daughter's death, she could tell the story of her daughter's life.

By telling the story of her daughter's life, from birth through her preschool and school years and including the death, what she accomplished was putting it all into language. Language, for adults, is processed in the left hemisphere because it is routine. She was able to shift enough of the emotional trauma locked in the limbic system to the left hemisphere, and she was able to begin to grieve.

She stated that on the very day she told the story of her daughter's life she had the dream again, only this time it did not end with her waking up as the gunman pulled the trigger. This time she saw him pull the trigger and shoot her daughter. This time she saw her daughter fall to the ground and die. But in her dream she went to her daughter, took her daughter's hand, and told her daughter how much she loved her and missed her. This woman was now able to grieve. She could now think about all the other memories of her daughter . . . the preschool years, the pictures she brought home that they hung on the refrigerator, the birthday parties, etc. She could revisit the healing memories, and she could grieve.

That is what good counseling is all about. It is not about giving advice. It is about listening to the client, but not merely listening. It is about being astute enough to ask the right questions . . . the questions that get the client to put into words, into language, those issues that the individual has not processed. It allows them to start to grieve their losses, and losses are not just about death. Losses include divorce, loss of friendships, loss of relationships, people leaving home, loss of esteem, loss of confidence, loss of the feeling that the world is a safe and orderly place, and on and on. All such losses have to be grieved to some extent, and the way we help people grieve those losses is to help them move some of the emotional trauma to the left hemisphere by utilizing the routine of language.

The same is true when we have a student who dies. I recall one incident when a very likeable and very popular eighth grade student died from a skateboard accident. We knew that the following day we would have lots of students in trauma. How do we help them? We provide opportunities to talk, but the key is how to present that opportunity.

What we do not do is ask, "How do you feel about John's death?" Most children will reply that they don't know or they don't want to talk about it. That does not get them to open up.

What we ask instead is, "How did you meet John? What is your favorite memory of John? What is your funniest memory of John?" Those questions are easier to answer because they are accessing episodic memory, but what they accomplish is getting the child to put their feelings into language. This allows them to move from trauma into grief. That is the best way to help them . . . to get them to begin the grieving process.

The same is true if you ever deal with a child with autism. When a child with autism has their routine disrupted, what happens? They may cry or tantrum, or they may run. For those who have worked in schools, if you have ever chased a child who was a "runner," you know what I mean. Does their reaction sound like fight or flight? That is exactly what they are experiencing. They are in fight or flight because their routine was disrupted.

The best way to calm these children down, to get them back on track, is to talk about their routines and get them back into their routines. The reason such a child has their own set of routine or ritualistic behavior is because it calms them. By getting them back into their routines we are actually shifting the locus of control out of the limbic system and back into the left hemisphere.

The fact that we now know that the locus of control can shift in our brains, and that performing routine tasks will result in the locus of control shifting to the left hemisphere, means that we can use that information to shift the locus of control at will. We can also teach children to do this. That skill can help them in sports and in competitions of all kinds, but more importantly it can be used to calm them when they are stressed.

We will discuss some techniques for doing just that in the following chapter. But before we can get to that it is important to understand habitual thought patterns and mindset and the roles that these can have in either causing, exacerbating, and/or in alleviating stress.

What are habitual thought patterns? Habitual thought patterns are simply the habits that we have in relation to how we think. We all have habits. We all have many, many habits that we are not aware of. Try this. Cross your arms over your chest. Now, cross them the other way. Whichever arm is on top, move it to the bottom and tuck the other hand under the opposite arm. Can you do it? How does it feel? Does it feel strange? That is because the way we cross our arms is a habit.

The habits that we have are not necessarily bad, although some of them might be, but our habits help us get through the day. We also have habits in the way we think about things. Again, these are not necessarily bad. In fact, we need them. If we really had to think through all the tasks we perform each day we would have real trouble getting much done. Problems occur, however, because some of those habitual thought patterns may be negative, or destructive, or even debilitating.

When we think about how the brain works we realize it is an amazing organ for learning. As we learn we forge neural pathways. Dendrites will bush out as learning progresses. The brain is a phenomenal organ at learning, but not so well equipped to unlearn what has been learned.

Have you ever gone back, as an adult, to visit your parents and your mother says something or does something and you are suddenly caught up in thoughts, reactions, and feelings that you had when you were a teenager? You are suddenly responding to her like you were thirteen?

Or have you ever gone back to a family gathering at Christmas, Chanukah, or Thanksgiving and your brother or sister said something or did something and you find yourself squabbling with them like you did when you were in middle school? Why do these things happen? It is because those neural pathways that were forged back then are still there. They have not gone away. Something happened to trigger those memories, and you are right back there in the thick of it with all the emotions, all the gut level responses, all the behaviors and mannerisms from long ago.

This is why habits are so hard to break. Understanding that the brain is great at forging neural pathways, at learning, but is not good at unlearning is important. It means that to change a habit it is best to learn a different habit rather than try to unlearn an old one. For example, if we are dieting and feeling hungry it is easier to learn to drink more water rather than to try not to eat food. Learning a different behavior is easier than unlearning an existing one. It is easier to learn to do something rather than learn not to do something.

Daniel Amen wrote a book for children called *Mind Coach* (2002). Amen discusses what he calls "automatic negative thoughts" that children have. These include "all or nothing" thinking, which means thinking that circumstances are either all good or all bad. There is no middle ground. There are no grey areas. People are good or bad, right or wrong. In reality there are a lot of grey areas in life.

A second automatic thought is "always" thinking. This is thinking that things are always one way, that I am always last, that I never get a turn, that life is always unfair. Some children see the world this way.

Then there is "focusing only on the negative." Some children can only seem to look at what is wrong in a situation . . . they cannot focus on anything that is right or that is going well. They cannot enjoy success because they know that failure is just around the corner, and they are thinking about that upcoming failure.

Another automatic negative thought involves "fortune telling." Children who practice this know what the future will be, and it will be bad. They can predict their own failure, they know that others won't like them, they know that things won't go well for them.

There are also children who practice "mind reading." They think they know what others think. They know that others think they are stupid, or that others think that what they are wearing is ugly. Rather than giving people the chance to respond to them openly and honestly, they think that others think the worst.

"Thinking with feelings" is another negative thought children sometimes practice. They tend to think that what they feel is correct without ever challenging those feelings. They let whatever feelings they have dictate what they say and what they do. Their feelings are in total control.

"Guilt beating" is another automatic negative way of thinking that children demonstrate. They think in terms like "I should," "I must," "I ought," and so forth. They are always feeling guilty about the better way they should have acted or responded.

"Labeling" is another negative thought pattern. Labeling refers to both labeling others and labeling oneself. Someone makes a mistake and we label them as stupid or dumb. Children also do that to themselves. They make a mistake and automatically start calling themselves stupid or dumb, saying things to themselves like, "I am just stupid," "I'm an idiot," "I am a dope."

The final negative thought Dr. Amen discusses is that of "blaming" others. That means that whatever goes wrong is someone else's fault. It means not taking the responsibility for one's actions on oneself, but rather pushing it off on others. The first step in managing one's behavior is to accept responsibility for what one did. If we don't own the behavior we will never be able to control it.

While these are automatic negative thoughts that Dr. Amen discusses in relation to children, it is also true that adults can have these automatic negative thought patterns. Habitually thinking in any of these ways can be very destructive to us and to our relationships with others.

Another aspect of habitual thinking is captured in the term "mindset." Carol Dweck wrote a book called *Mindset* (2006). Mindset refers to the way we think about our abilities or our intelligence. Is our level of intelligence set, or can it change. . .can it grow? Everyone thinks one way or the other. We either think that how smart we are is set in stone, or we think that we can get smarter by what we do, by what we learn, by diligent effort. The way we think about this greatly determines how we act . . . how we lead our lives. Many people lead "lives of quiet desperation" as the saying goes. Those are people with a fixed mindset.

In her book, Dweck discusses a simple study done with seventh grade students. These students were asked questions to determine whether they had a fixed or a growth mindset. Once that was determined, the researchers simply watched the math scores of these two groups over the next two years. The group of students that had the growth mindset surpassed the fixed mindset group in math performance.

Since mindset had a measurable impact on math performance, they went back to an incoming group of seventh grade students to do an experiment. They went to those students who were already showing difficulties in math and divided them into two groups.

The first group was given a study skills course, just like the study skills courses often given to students who are struggling. The second group was given a short course in how the brain works. They were taught that we forge neural pathways as we learn. They were taught that dendrites bush out to allow the brain to communicate faster and better as things become stronger in our memories . . . in our learning. They were taught that we actually change our brain and change how it functions as we learn. After these groups finished their respective courses, the math grades were again watched for two years. The group that had been taught about the brain, that had been taught a growth mindset, surpassed the other group in math performance.

What happens with mindset is this; the fixed mindset displays an urgency to prove itself over and over. If we believe our attributes are set, that our intelligence is set, then we are always on trial. We are always being judged, we are always being measured, and we must continually prove our worth. All of our actions become an intelligence test . . . an abilities test. If we believe that we cannot prove our worth, that we cannot measure up, then we will soon stop trying. Every task becomes about succeeding or failing rather than about learning and growing.

The growth mindset, on the other hand, is all about learning and growing. The growth mindset starts with the notion that the hand we are dealt is the starting point, not the ending point of our intelligence and our abilities. Where can we go from here? The growth mindset is about development while the fixed mindset is about validation.

Our mindset also significantly impacts the effort we put into things. In the fixed mindset world effort becomes a negative thing. If we were really smart, really talented, we would not have to try so hard. We can hear this fixed mindset in schools all the time. Some students will get an "A" on a test but you can hear them say things like, "I hardly even studied," "I barely even looked at my notes," "I didn't crack the book." After all, if they were truly smart they wouldn't have to study. Admitting they studied would be like admitting they weren't smart. We can hear other students say things like, "I really worked hard for that test, I studied my tail off." That is a growth mindset talking.

Unfortunately what we too often see with students who have a fixed mindset, even students who really are quite capable, is that they will drop out. We see students who breeze through elementary school, middle school, and high school, but then enter college and the competition is tougher. They look around and don't think they can measure up, so they drop out. The growth mindset student would look around and determine that they just need to work harder, but the fixed mindset student will leave school. They don't believe that they could do the work if they really tried . . . if they really put forth the effort.

That is a big adjustment for a lot of students entering college, and that is why some turn around and go home. Some students drop out much earlier than that. Some drop out in high school, and some drop out mentally in middle school or even elementary school. How many of those physical or mental dropouts could we turn around if we addressed their mindset?

The mindset that we have can be seen even as early as four years old. There was another study reported by Dweck that looked at four year olds. These children were asked questions to determine whether they had a fixed mindset or a growth mindset, and then they were allowed to play with jigsaw puzzles. After mastering the puzzles they were given an option . . . they could either continue to play with the same puzzles, or they could play with some new ones. The new ones were harder puzzles, they had more pieces. The students were shown the new puzzles so they could see that they were harder.

What happened was that the fixed mindset children wanted to continue to play with the same puzzles they had been playing with; they had already proven themselves on these puzzles. The growth mindset children wanted the new puzzles. They wanted a shot at a new challenge. The mindset that these children had determined their willingness to tackle new tasks. How often do we see that in students?

It seems that for a fixed mindset individual, when they fail at something, it invalidates them. In school we sometimes see very good students, students who make top grades on everything they do, but they have this fixed mindset. What often happens is that they are terrified of not doing well on a test. They over-study for tests to the point that they become nervous wrecks. They are afraid to fail because it would invalidate them permanently. All the past successes don't matter. One failure and they are proven to be a charlatan, a faker. Failure is transformed from an action, I failed, to an identity, I'm a failure. Know any students like that?

Yet another study Dweck reported was one with adolescents. They were working difficult problems and at some point the researchers began to praise the students. Some students were praised by telling them that they were doing a great job and they must be smart. Another group was praised by telling them that they were doing a great job and they were putting forth great effort. In other words, some students were pushed toward a fixed mindset by telling them they were smart, while other students were pushed toward a growth mindset by praising their effort.

Almost immediately differences were noticed. The fixed mindset students were more reluctant to continue. They had already proven themselves to be smart and the only way to go from there was down . . . so why continue? The growth mindset students had no problem continuing. The level of work also deteriorated for the fixed mindset students. They had been told they were smart, so if they did not continue to do well they would prove they were not smart. Hence they began feeling pressure or stress. More precisely, they were experiencing a threat to ego. With the introduction of stress into the equation for the fixed mindset students, the quality of their work declined.

Mindset is again a part of habitual thought patterns. It is the habitual way we think about things, especially our own abilities. We can address that in children and by doing so build a growth mindset which would be ever so much more productive and less stress producing in their lives. The charge and task of educating children would be so much easier if we understand and utilize these concepts.

## Chapter 9

# Improving Sleep

## Some Basic Techniques for Stress Reduction

*What is the difference between cats and dogs? There is a book called* Cat and Dog Theology *(Sjogren 2005), which addresses this question. A dog looks at you and thinks, "You feed me, you water me, you shelter me, you pet me, you take care of me, you must be God." And the dog is devoted to you. A cat looks at you and thinks, "You feed me, you water me, you shelter me, you pet me, you take care of me, I must be God." And the cat is devoted to itself. The difference is in focus.*

*This focus is important in how we look at life, how we look at religion, and how we look at others. When I look at you, are you important to me, or is it all about me? When someone has a focus that life is all about themselves and their own needs, and others are basically there to be used, the resulting relationships become meaningless and are easily discarded. What is the focus we bring to life?*

In the last chapter we discussed stress, what stress is all about, what causes stress, what happens in the brain when we experience stress, and a little about how the brain functions so we can better understand stress. Now we want to discuss how to manage stress. In the following chapter we will discuss specific ways to improve sleep, both the quality and quantity of sleep. In this chapter we will specifically discuss managing stress because that also impacts how we sleep.

Stress impacts us in multiple ways, but the focus of this book is on sleep, so we will attempt to limit the discussion of stress management and stress reduction to the impact that has on sleep. Please keep in mind that children and adolescents face a great deal of stress but they have not had many life experiences that help them know how to manage it. Consequently, it is crucial that we make the effort to teach children how to manage stress because it has the potential to significantly impact the sleep they get.

Some key points we will focus on include the use of routine to actually shift the locus of control in the brain, the importance of addressing habitual thought patterns and how we can do that, and the value of creating an outward focus as opposed to an overabundance of introspection. If we can help children learn these things they can reduce the daily stress they experience.

To begin with, how can we utilize routine in our favor? We have discussed how routine functions are controlled in the left hemisphere and how doing routine things or thinking routine thoughts will actually shift the locus of control. We can use that knowledge to hit better golf shots, but we can also use it to reduce stress at any specific time. To use routine, however, you must first build routine. There are a number of practices or disciplines that teach and utilize routine as an integral part of their process. These would include such practices as yoga, tai chi, biofeedback, relaxation techniques, meditation, or deep breathing.

Yoga was developed as part of a religious, meditative experience. In the western world it is mainly used as a system of exercise that utilizes routine postures, routine slow breathing, and meditation.

The routine of yoga is calming. It slows us down, it lowers our blood pressure and heart rates. Practicing some yoga postures at the end of a stressful day can have a very beneficial effect on our stress level. Teaching yoga to children who have anger issues, who are nervous, or who exhibit high stress can be a very positive tool. When they experience stress or anger we can remind them to use their yoga skills and, through these skills, they can learn to manage their own stress rather than rely on us to manage it for them. That is the ultimate goal for children. . .to give them the tools to manage their own emotions and emotional experiences.

Tai chi is another practice that utilizes routine. Tai chi was developed in China and is considered a martial art, but it is considered deflective rather than aggressive. It uses gentle, controlled, and routine movements that flow from one pose to another. While yoga strives for routine poses that are held for periods of time, tai chi utilizes a continuous, fluid movement from pose to pose and through the poses. Again, however, using the routine of tai chi after a stressful day can lower our stress level, and using tai chi or yoga on a regular basis can help us maintain a lowered stress level. And, like yoga, tai chi can be taught to children to help them manage stress.

Biofeedback is yet another tool at our disposal. The term biofeedback was developed in the late 1960s when it was used to help subjects get in touch with the physiological responses they were experiencing, and learn to alter those responses. The responses included such things as blood pressure, heart rate, perspiration, muscle tension, etc. The individual receives feedback regarding these physiological responses and learns to alter them through breathing and concentration. By doing so an individual can lower his or her stress level. There are offices where adults or children can go to learn biofeedback techniques, and there are also sites where people can buy equipment for using biofeedback at home.

Using one of multiple types of relaxation techniques is also a great way to relieve stress. Relaxation techniques include autogenic relaxation, progressive muscle relaxation, and visualization techniques. Autogenic refers to something that comes from within us or inside us. An autogenic technique, therefore, would use our own visual imagery and/or body awareness to decrease stress. We might repeat certain words or certain phrases to ourselves, or we might repeat suggestions to ourselves that help us relax and reduce the tightness in our bodies . . . in our muscles. We might use our imaginations to picture a specific peaceful place or setting we know as we focus on controlling and relaxing our breathing and our heart rate or our pulse rate. Or we might focus on relaxing specific parts of our bodies.

In progressive muscle relaxation we would focus on slowly tensing and then relaxing each set of muscles. We might start by first tensing then relaxing the muscles in our toes and feet. After a few moments with toes and feet, we might turn to the ankles and calves. Then we move up to the thighs, then the buttocks. Then we might tense and relax the muscles in the lower back. We would do the same with our fingers and hands, then our forearms, then our biceps. Finally we would tense and relax the muscles in our neck and then in our ears and the side of our head, and finally we would tense and relax our facial muscles around our mouth, our eyes, and our forehead. With each set of muscles we would tense them for five to ten seconds and then relax them for about thirty seconds.

This technique helps us to focus on the difference in our body between tension and relaxation states. It helps us to be aware of our bodily sensations. This is a great technique not only to reduce stress but to put ourselves to sleep. There are also tapes and CDs that can be purchased that will take us through this progressive muscle relaxation.

Visualization is a technique in which we form mental images and take a visual journey to a peaceful or calming place. Visualization, while implying visual imagery, can effectively utilize many of our senses in this process. We certainly use the visual images, but along with that if we can imagine smells and aromas, pleasant sounds, pleasing textures and tactile sensations, our imagery will be more powerful and more relaxing.

For example, if the seashore is a relaxing place for us, we might imagine the sight of the ocean and the waves crashing on the shoreline, we might imagine the sun rising or setting over the water, we might imagine the sound of the waves as they meet the shore, we might smell the ocean scents, we might feel the warmth of the sun on our face or feel the sensation of the sand between our toes. You get the picture. To use visualization effectively we need to close our eyes, loosen any tight clothing, and sit or lie in a comfortable position away from noise or other distractions.

Music can also be used as a relaxation technique. The music needs to be calming music, however, not rap music, or hip hop, or heavy metal, or anything that is fast paced or that changes in tempo or in volume. It should also be instrumental music rather than vocal music. If we use vocal music we can get caught up in the words and then the mind engages when what we want to happen is to let the mind drift.

Music that is really great for relaxing is the music often used for yoga. Such music is often called music for meditation. It is slow, quiet, and repetitive. Children and especially adolescents, however, may not be inclined to listen to the types of music that would be relaxing. Therefore, the use of music for relaxation may not be as effective for teens as it can be for adults.

Exercise is another relaxation technique that is helpful for some people. The exercise itself is invigorating and stimulating, but several hours after the exercise our heart rate and our breathing rate is lower and we reap the relaxation benefit. Hence exercise should be done earlier in the day, not right before going to bed. Regular exercise will help us become better at relaxing. It is also true that as we exercise vigorously enough to sweat, the act of sweating eliminates certain toxins from our bodies. We actually sweat out toxic substances, and that also enables and promotes better relaxation.

Using guided imagery is another great way to reduce stress. There are many tapes and CDs that use the techniques we discussed about visualization and progressive muscle relaxation. These can be wonderful tools to both help us relax and to help us go to sleep if we make a habit of using them. The first time someone uses such a CD or tape it might not be as effective as if they continue to use it. The routine thoughts we have when the words become common to us will eventually put us to sleep very quickly.

Any of these relaxation techniques can be taught to children as a means to reduce stress and/or as a means to manage sleep. What works for one child, however, may not be helpful to another, so trying different approaches might be necessary.

Yet another way to reduce stress is through meditation. Meditation is a component of many eastern religions, but it is also used by many people for non-religious reasons. It is used to relax, to find peace or quiescence, to focus attention and hype up mental concentration, or to achieve a higher state of consciousness. Meditation is basically the self-regulation of attention. It is a discipline in which the mind is focused on an object, a thought, a process, or an awareness. The different techniques of meditation are often classified based on their focus. There is "mindfulness" meditation and "concentrative" meditation.

In mindfulness meditation the meditator focuses on the field or background perceptions or experiences. The individual sits comfortably and silently and centers his attention by focusing his awareness on an object or a process. Such processes could be one's breath, a sound or mantra like "ohm," a koan that evokes a question, a visual image, a mental exercise like mentally untying a knot. The individual attempts to maintain an open focus allowing his mind to shift freely from one perception to another. No thought, image, or sensation is considered an intrusion, but the effort is to remain in the here and now, to stay in the present, to not think about the future or the past or fantasize about anything. The meditator continues to come back to the present and avoid cognitive analysis, using the focus of his perceptions as an anchor to the here and now.

Concentrative meditation is an effort to hold one's attention on a particular object, thought, or process while minimizing distractions. The meditator attempts to always come back to the specific object of attention, a candle, a mantra, an image, and so forth. Some forms of meditation combine both mindfulness and concentrative meditation. Whichever form of meditation is used takes some practice to get started. Once learned, however, meditation can have significant benefits in helping us to relax and de-stress our lives, and can be extremely beneficial for children and adolescents.

Deep breathing is another way to manage stress. Many people breathe shallowly. The telltale signs of shallow breathing are that the ribcage or the chest expands as we breathe. When we are anxious or stressed we tend to breathe shallowly. In fact, unnecessary tension in our muscles impedes our breathing. Deep breathing comes from the stomach. It is also referred to as diaphragmatic breathing, abdominal breathing, or belly breathing because when we breathe deeply the stomach rises and falls with each breath. Why is this important?

If we look at the mechanics involved in deep breathing we must note the diaphragm. The diaphragm is a structure that acts as a partition between our heart and lungs on the upper end, and other internal organs below. The diaphragm actually supports the heart. When we breathe deeply the diaphragm moves downward as we inhale and upward as we exhale. The more deeply we breathe the further the diaphragm moves in both directions. The more the diaphragm moves down during the inhalation stage the more our lungs are able to expand. Our lungs are actually larger at the bottom than at the top and deep breathing takes advantage of that. With this greater expansion the lungs can actually take in more oxygen, and during exhale release more carbon dioxide. This happens with each breath.

Besides this increase in oxygen and decrease in carbon dioxide, there are some other significant effects of deep breathing. First, when the diaphragm moves through this full range of motion with deep breathing it actually massages the organs. This moves fluid, known as lymphatic fluid, through the lymphatic system.

The lymphatic system is a complex network of lymphoid organs, lymph nodes, lymph ducts, lymphatic tissues, lymph capillaries, and lymph vessels. They function to carry lymph fluid to the circulatory system. The main functions of the lymphatic system are to remove excess fluids from our body tissues, to aid in the absorption of fatty acids and transport fat to the circulatory system, and to produce immune cells known as lymphocytes and monocytes.

Hence the lymphatic system is a major player in our immune system (Wikipedia 2001). Unlike the circulatory system that has a pump (the heart), the lymphatic system has no pump. It depends on muscle movement, on muscle massage to move the lymphatic fluids. Deep breathing acts as this massage to the organs and aids in the movement and function of the lymphatic system. When fluids are not moved properly we have swelling, or edema.

Another impact of the slower, deeper breathing and the rhythmical pumping of the diaphragm is that it helps engage our parasympathetic nervous system (The Fibromyalgia Community 1997). The parasympathetic system and the sympathetic system work together . . . they are complementary to each other. An analogy would be that the sympathetic system is like the accelerator on the car and the parasympathetic system is the brake. The sympathetic system initiates the fight-or-flight response and the parasympathetic system the relaxation-and-rest response. Deep breathing kicks in the parasympathetic system and thus aids in this relaxation response and hence reduces our stress levels.

To practice deep breathing it is important to have children sit down or lie down in a comfortable position, loosen any tight clothing so they don't feel constricted, place one hand on the stomach and the other hand on the chest, slowly inhale (don't gasp in air) and allow the stomach to rise and expand. Their hands can feel whether it is the stomach or the chest that is expanding. It must be the stomach. Then they slowly exhale, rest momentarily, and repeat the process. Many children, or adults for that matter, do not typically breathe deeply. With practice it can become the routine way we breathe.

A practice that I think is helpful with children is to practice "power breathing." The way to begin is to first have the children breathe like they are angry. Spend a little time having them practice this, and then briefly talk about what that was like. Then have them breathe like they are frightened. After doing that for a while discuss what that was like. Then have them all practice breathing like they are calm and in control. Discuss what that feels like.

After these exercises have a discussion that explains that the way we feel can and does impact the way we breathe, but the important thing to know is that it also works the other way around . . . the way we breathe impacts how we feel. In other words, if we are angry or frightened, but we intentionally breathe like we are calm and in control, we start to feel like we are calmer and more in control. Then we can have children imagine scenarios in which they are frightened or angry and practice breathing like they are calm and in control. This gives them the power to manage their emotions better and to lower their own stress level when they need to do so.

Another way to use routine to lower stress is to address how organized we are. Some adults are so disorganized that they can never find what they want. Every time they go somewhere they must first search for the car keys. Every task first involves searching for tools, trying to remember what they did with something, or how they can go about getting the information they need again because they cannot find what they once had. With children it might be finding their homework or finding their belt or shoes. Every task begins with chaos and stress. Their lives are in chaos because of their lack of organization. Reducing that chaos by learning some organizational skills can significantly lower stress.

Learning problem solving skills is another technique useful in managing stress. When something goes wrong in our lives what is our response? Do we fall apart? Some people do. . .some children do. Learning a systematic approach to problem solving means that when our world falls apart we don't have to follow suit. It means that we have a routine set of steps to follow that will help us make a decision about what to do next. That routine gives us time to evaluate rather than react. It gives us the chance to resolve the problem rather than go into fight or flight because of the problem.

Teaching children a problem-solving routine gives them control over their negative emotions, and gives them the opportunity to respond rather than react. If all a child has in his arsenal is reaction, that is stressful . . . and that often leads to further stress just around the corner . . . the stress that comes from their poor reaction to the initial stress.

What are the critical steps in problem solving? There are different methods that are used, and some of us might prefer one method over another, but there are some basic concepts that any method should include. This includes asking ourselves some basic questions, and then following some basic steps.

There are three questions that are critical. First, what assumptions are we making about this problem or this issue? We all make assumptions. We do it all the time. We need assumptions, but sometimes they get in our way. So what assumptions are we making as opposed to what facts we really know? Knowing something for sure as a fact is one thing, but if it is only an assumption we must look at the accuracy or potential inaccuracy of the assumption and our reaction to it. We need to articulate these assumptions either verbally or in writing so we are clear.

Second, what resources are there that might help us with the problem or issue? These resources, usually other people, can be utilized at any time. They are especially valuable early on because other people can give another perspective on the issue that we had not considered.

Third, can the problem be broken down into smaller segments? Sometimes problems can seem overwhelming . . . so overwhelming that we are immobilized. If we can break it down into smaller segments, the problem becomes more manageable.

After considering those three questions, and any further questions those questions might bring, we must look at the process of solving the problem or its parts. The first step is to look at the last step. What outcome do we want? How do we want this to end?

In teaching this to children we should have them write that down on one side of a piece of paper, say the left side. Draw a box around it. Next have them think about and write down on the right side of the paper all the possible choices they could make. Write them down and number them, regardless of how good a decision they think each might be. This is called brainstorming the possible choices. It is important to brainstorm options because if we have only one option . . . that is not a choice. We need multiple options to really have a choice.

After the child writes down all of the options, he needs to think about what result each of these options is likely to achieve. Are any of the children likely to achieve what they want? Are any of them likely to achieve what they have written in the box on the left side of the paper? For those options that have that potential, they should draw a line from that option to the box.

Now that they have choices, or have limited their choices, they can make a decision as to what they are going to do. They now have an informed decision. They now have a plan that has some possibility of being successful because they didn't react but rather responded. The final act in problem solving is to evaluate the outcome. Did they achieve their goal? If they did not then maybe they need to begin again, or again seek assistance from other resources.

Teaching children such a problem solving process lowers their stress level. Whether it works every time or not, it still keeps them calmer and keeps them from flying off the handle. It keeps them from gong into fight or flight when fight or flight is not really a necessary or appropriate response.

Another key in managing or reducing stress is to look at habitual thought patterns. As we mentioned in the last chapter, habitual thought patterns are the habitual ways we think about things. When we have habitual thoughts that are stress producing we need to find ways to change those thoughts. That is accomplished by first articulating the negative thoughts that we have, and then replacing those thoughts with other, more positive, more productive thoughts.

Let's look at some examples. One common thought that a lot of people face has to do with their weight. We struggle with our weight. We try to lose weight but cannot seem to do it. We make a little headway and drop a few pounds and then we go and undermine our success with an episode of binging. Sound familiar?

If we examine our thoughts we might begin to notice that we are having very negative thoughts about ourselves. We are thinking things like, "I'm just a fat pig, I'll never look good, I have no will power, I'm fat . . . fat . . . fat, I don't deserve to look good because I can't control myself, I deserve a treat," and on and on. This habitual thinking does not help us to lose weight and, in fact, is one of the reasons we do not lose weight. The habitual thoughts we are having keep us from being successful at losing weight.

To deal with this we first must examine the thoughts we are having, and write them down. Then we must decide on thoughts that are more positive . . . thoughts that can really help us achieve our goal of weight loss. We definitely need to write these down and use them as affirmations. They might include such thoughts as, "I will lose weight, I can do this, I am worth the effort, Deep down I am a thin person just waiting to come out, I will reward my small victories in a positive manner rather than undermining myself for the victories, I am worth loving and I will love myself first."

The next step is to read these affirmations every morning and every evening. We read them until we can recite them in our sleep. We read them until they are a part of us, until these thoughts . . . these affirmations . . . ooze from our pores. These affirmations, these positive thoughts have to become our habitual thoughts.

Please understand that this is not advocating that we need to lose weight or to be thin to be happy or to like ourselves. The point is that if this is something we want, then the way to achieve it is to have positive thoughts about ourselves and our goals. Those positive affirmations must replace the negative thoughts. It isn't enough to merely try to avoid the negative thoughts. We must replace them with positive thoughts, and practice those positive thoughts every day.

Another example is road rage. Road rage does not just happen. It occurs because we allow certain negative thinking to enter our minds about what other drivers are doing to us, or inflicting on us, or how they are disrespecting us. These habitual negative thoughts build to the point that eventually someone cuts in front of us and we are automatically in a rage.

Again, to effectively deal with this we need to first examine and articulate the thoughts that we are having. Then we need to replace that habitual thinking with more positive thoughts. This could include such thoughts as, "That driver may be an idiot for driving dangerously, but he is not doing it as disrespect to me. It has nothing to do with me. I will not allow his driving actions to control my day. I am worth more than that. I will be in control of my emotions. I will not abdicate control of my emotions to that other driver. I will not be late because of him. I will be just fine and I will have a great day."

These are obviously just examples. The specific affirmations one needs will depend somewhat on the negative thinking they have been having. The point is, if we read the positive affirmations every day so that they become our habitual thoughts, that will help us to overcome road rage.

While the examples given for addressing negative or unproductive thoughts or thought patterns have concerned weight loss or road rage, these same techniques can be applied to any negative thinking that we find ourselves engaging in. This negative thinking is often at the root of stress for children and adolescents, and we can help them lower their stress or manage their stress better if they attack the negative habitual thinking that they too often allow themselves to have. We can teach them to create and practice positive affirmations and positive thought patterns.

Yet another way to lower stress or manage stress is to create an outward focus. Too often we look inside ourselves, we practice introspection, we get so caught up in looking at our own situation that we fail to put it in perspective. Children and adolescents do this all the time. This belly button gazing, if that is all they do, elevates their stress.

To be healthy certainly involves doing some self-evaluation, but it also involves looking outside ourselves. Having an outward focus opens children to building connections with others. It opens them to being able to understand others and feel empathy for their plight. It helps them find their place in the world. They really cannot achieve those things by only looking inside. Learning to focus outside rather than inside does not diminish them, but it helps them see themselves from a different perspective. Having a broader perspective about life diminishes the stress that they feel about their own lives.

An outward focus can be achieved by volunteering, by doing something to help another individual or group of individuals. Helping a child find what he has to offer others can help him realize the blessings that he has. It can change his perspective from one of looking merely at his deficits, at his problems, to one of seeing what he really does possess in his life. The old saying, "I felt bad that I had no shoes until I saw a man who had no feet," is very applicable. This is not a Pollyanna approach. Getting involved with other people, with the world outside of one's inner sanctum, will change one's own perspective.

This also goes back to the dog and cat theology that was cited at the beginning of this chapter. Those who view the world from the cat perspective, that they are the only thing of importance, that everyone and everything they encounter is merely for their own pleasure, are significantly impacted when little things go wrong with their world. Those who have more of the dog outlook, that others are also important, have a different perspective. They don't tend to get so caught up in their own problems. Problems are seen in a broader perspective and become less relevant in the scheme of things.

When we look at individuals who are depressed, do they have an outward focus or are they mainly focused inside at their own issues? Certainly one important means of stress management is to see things from a different perspective . . . to focus outside ourselves.

One final way of lowering stress is to talk things out. Get into the habit of talking things out. Men and boys are typically very poor at this. They look at a problem and want a solution, and if they don't think that others can give them a solution they don't want to waste time talking the issue over with anyone else. That is the wrong way to think!

Talking a problem out is not about getting advice. It is not about having someone else provide a solution. Talking a problem out is about putting that problem into language. Language is a left hemisphere activity (for adolescents and adults) and putting issues into language moves those issues to the left hemisphere. It allows the individual with the problem or issue to begin to grieve it, to put it in the perspective of past experiences, to process it, and to possibly come to some decisions about the problem.

When an individual talks things out he will often solve the problem for himself, or at least find a way to come to terms with the problem. It is not that the listener is doing anything to help . . . other than being a listener. It is the very act of putting the problem into language that helps the individual deal with the problem, and by dealing with such problems they lower their stress. That is certainly more productive than going into a cave when a problem arises, as is the practice of many males and, yes, some females. Teaching children and adolescents the value of talking about problems is a valuable tool in helping them both solve and/or reduce stress.

Managing stress is certainly an important aspect of allowing us to function better and to sleep better, and it is crucial that we teach this to children. Now let's turn to more specific ways to improve sleep.

*Chapter 10*

# Specific Strategies for Improving the Quantity and Quality of Sleep

## Using the Senses

*At 211° water is hot . . . very hot. At 212° it boils. This is pointed out very well in the book* 212°-The Extra Degree *by Sam Parker and Mac Anderson (2006). That one degree makes a huge difference. When water boils it makes steam, and with steam comes the ability to power a locomotive. One degree can make all the difference in the world. The same is true of the sleep we get. One or two very subtle, very minor changes in what we do can make all the difference. That one extra degree of difference, of effort, can make a one hundred and eighty degree impact in our lives.*

How can we improve the quality and the quantity of sleep? We have attempted to make the point throughout this book that this is a very worthwhile and necessary goal, but how can we achieve that goal? One of the first steps is to realize that all sleep is not necessarily quality sleep. Many people wake up from a night of sleep and they feel fatigued, exhausted, and certainly not rested. This can happen with people suffering from fibromyalgia, post-traumatic stress disorder, or depression.

What do these conditions have in common? First of all, stress is a common precipitating factor. Some studies, for example, have concluded that fibromyalgia is linked to post-traumatic stress disorder (Wikipedia 2001). Secondly, slow wave sleep is also disrupted in all of these conditions. Slow wave sleep is the deep, restful sleep, but also the sleep stage during which growth hormone is released. Without sufficient slow wave sleep we are both exhausted and can have physical pain.

People suffering from depression also get less slow wave sleep, but unlike fibromyalgia or PTSD it is because they are getting an overabundance of REM sleep. REM sleep is very necessary for processing emotional issues, but it is also exhausting. The brain is very active during REM sleep. If we get too much REM and not enough slow wave, we also wake up exhausted. How many adolescents do you know who seem both depressed and fatigued?

People who suffer from sleep apnea, and to a lesser extent people who are heavy snorers, also tend to not get enough slow wave sleep. Sleep apnea, which is a stoppage of breathing followed by a gasping for breath, keeps the individual from progressing into slow wave sleep. The oxygen deprivation, the constant gasping for air, causes them to linger in levels one and two of non-REM sleep, which are the stages nearest to wakefulness. Besides the health issues related to sleep apnea, those with this condition are also not as well rested as they should be after sleep.

What else can keep us from going into the restful slow wave sleep? Pain can do it. If we are waking regularly because of pain we will not be getting as much slow wave sleep. Restless leg syndrome, where the legs just keep jumping and twitching will result in less slow wave sleep. Prostate problems or frequent urinary urges can keep us from getting slow wave sleep. Headaches, hormonal changes, hot flashes, heartburn, allergies, or asthma can also prevent us from getting enough slow wave sleep.

Some over-the-counter medications can also decrease our ability to go into or remain in slow wave sleep. Some illicit drugs will do that. Caffeine, alcohol, or tobacco can have this effect. Again, how many teens do you know who smoke, drink alcohol, and/or regularly use high-caffeine drinks?

Having nightmares regularly or being under sufficient stress that we keep waking with issues on our minds can also keep us from slow wave sleep.

With adolescents especially, considering all the things that can keep them from getting enough slow wave, restful sleep, it is not surprising that we have so many adolescents who awaken from sleep and are still exhausted. All is not lost, however. There are many things that can be done to improve sleep. Let's begin with sleep apnea. Children or adolescents with sleep apnea, or even heavy snoring, are most likely not getting the quality rest they need. This should be addressed. I would strongly recommend seeing a physician or going to a sleep clinic to address this issue.

Remember, anything that restricts the oxygen flow in the upper air passage can result in snoring or sleep apnea. Being overweight can cause this, so losing weight will help. Drinking alcohol can cause this because it relaxes the muscles and lets them sag, thus restricting the air passage . . . so avoiding alcohol before bed can help. This is just one of many reasons why adolescents should not drink alcohol. Learning to sleep on one's side rather than on one's back can help avoid this air restriction. It has been suggested that exercising the muscles of the throat and neck might help because toning these muscles can keep them from sagging, thus promoting better air flow.

For children or adolescents who are suffering from depression, it is important to address and try to resolve the issues that are depressing them. Taking Prozac or other anti-depressant medications are not recommended for youth, and these medications do not address the issues that are causing the depression anyway. Those issues must be addressed.

For those who wake up at night because of all the stress in their lives and find themselves just lying there with all the troublesome thoughts racing through their heads, it is important to try to separate those thoughts from sleep. Teach children and adolescents to set aside a time to think about those issues. For example, set aside an hour earlier in the evening to think about the problems and the worries they have. Then, an hour before bed, do something restful to wind down. Then go to bed. Make that a routine and it will start to be a cue to the brain and body that sleep is imminent.

It may also be helpful to teach adolescents to write down the troublesome issues on a sheet of paper and set them aside, physically and symbolically, with the thought that they will deal with these issues tomorrow. That can work before bed, but it can also be done if adolescents awaken during the night with problems on their minds.

Some other steps to take to help children get to sleep, or get back to sleep, would involve the senses. Although we now know there are more than five senses, let's talk about the sense of sight, the sense of smell, the sense of hearing, the sense of taste, and the sense of touch. It is helpful to think about sleep strategies in terms of these five senses because it helps not to overlook something that might be significant for a child. These senses can keep us awake and/or awaken us, but they can also be used to help us go to sleep.

The sense of sight is the first and foremost sense we must address. To sleep we must close our eyes. Trying to doze off while watching television is not a good way to get to sleep. It can be done, especially if we finally get tired enough, but we miss a lot of beneficial sleep by getting into that habit and are more than likely sleep deprived. This is a very poor habit for teens to develop. Ideally the bedroom, or wherever they sleep, should be free from televisions, computers, or other such clutter. The visuals are distracting.

It is also important to sleep in darkness. Even with our eyes closed we can detect light, and that can keep us awake and disrupt melatonin release. Some children have nightmares and they want a night light to make them feel safer. In those situations a light may be the lesser of two evils, but for adolescents it is far better to sleep in darkness. That light that is left on when they go to sleep may be the very reason they awaken at two-thirty in the morning. That could be the hallway light or the light from the television. It also might be helpful to dim the lights in the house or in their rooms about an hour or so before going to bed as a signal to the body that rest is coming and to start shutting down and preparing for sleep.

Besides dimming the lights in the evening, it is also important to expose adolescents to bright light in the morning. Exposure to bright light in the morning helps the circadian rhythm to adjust the sleep-wake cycles. So we should throw open the drapes and have our adolescent face the sunlight when he first gets up. That simple act in the morning will help put him to sleep at night.

A second sense that we need to address to improve sleep would be the sense of hearing. We sleep best when it is quiet. Again, that means it is not wise to go to sleep with the television on. We may eventually drift off to sleep with it on, but there is also the very likely possibility that it will awaken us later on in the evening. The habit of going to sleep with the television on is a great way to build up sleep deprivation in adolescents.

Some adolescents claim they need a little noise as a distraction to help them sleep. If that is the case, try music instead of the television. The music should be quiet, calm, and repetitive music. Listening to rock music, rap, or something with a driving beat, or something that changes tempo or changes in volume is not restful. It will have just the opposite impact.

If the choice of music becomes a real issue, then go with a CD or tape of guided imagery or relaxation instead. There are relaxation CDs that coach us into progressively relaxing one part of the body at a time, or guided imagery CDs that help us sleep by taking us to a quiet, restful place in our imaginations. Having the adolescent listen to these will eventually put him to sleep rather quickly. He will get used to the sound of the same repetitive voice, the same instructions, and that repetition eventually has a hypnotic effect and the mind drifts off to sleep fairly quickly.

Using the sense of touch, the tactile sensations, is also a good way to assist in the quest for improved sleep. This can take several different forms. Having a massage certainly relaxes the muscles and is a sleep aid, but that is not often practical. A little self-massage is. Rub the sore muscles, or the places that are aching. This might also include a little light stretching before bed to stretch out and relax any tightness or soreness in the body.

Using the tactile senses also means making sure we feel clean before bed. Encourage an adolescent to take a shower or, even better, a warm bath before bed. Then rub on some light oil or lotion. Brushing our teeth so that the mouth feels clean is also important. Brushing the mouth not only cleanses it but also removes any lingering tastes from whatever was eaten that evening.

When there are sleep problems a little something in the stomach is also helpful. Provide a light snack for adolescents before bed. Going to bed with an empty stomach can keep them awake. Likewise, going to bed with a really full stomach can keep them awake because of the tightness and discomfort. Having just a light snack is optimal. Additionally, going to bed with a little something in the stomach draws blood to the stomach for digestion, and hence away from the brain. That also promotes sleep.

While a light snack may aid sleep, a lot of fluids before bed should be avoided. Fluids will cause the adolescent to awaken within a few hours to urinate, and if there are problems getting back to sleep, then the entire sleep effort can be undermined.

Another facet of using tactile senses involves the heat or coolness of the body. One of the functions of going to sleep is that our bodies cool down. This natural drop in temperature helps us go to sleep (Martin 2002, 94). In the morning before we wake up, if we awaken naturally rather than by an alarm clock, our body temperature starts to rise. This is part of the waking cycle.

We often use this without even realizing it. Taking a warm bath feels good to our skin and relaxes us, but a part of what is happening is related to heat and coolness. The heat of the bath warms us, but then when we get out of the bath we start to cool off, and the relative cooling off is a part of what helps us to sleep.

The same is true when we drink a cup of warm milk before bed. Milk contains both tryptophan and calcium. Tryptophan, with the aid of calcium, can be converted to melatonin in our bodies, which is important in sleep. However, the actual warmth of the milk also plays a critical part. The warm milk warms us up, and then as we cool off afterwards the relative cooling off puts us to sleep.

Knowing this, it is important to manage the temperature appropriately before bed. Encourage adolescents to avoid covering up so much that they are toasty, especially if they are having trouble sleeping. Have you ever noticed on a hot summer's evening when the air conditioning has broken down and you are lying there feeling very hot, that it is incredibly difficult to get to sleep? In fact, the optimal ambient temperature for nocturnal sleeping is between 65–68 degrees. Body temperature is an important sleep factor.

For adolescents who are having trouble sleeping, they should be slightly cool. Turn the thermostat down to a cooler temperature. That will help them to drift off. Also they should try to cool off before climbing into bed. In the winter this is easy. Have them step out on the back porch for a few minutes before going to bed. Cooling down the body significantly and then climbing into a comfortable bed will often put them right to sleep.

If they awaken during the night, this same strategy can be useful. For those who awaken at night and find it difficult to return to sleep . . . have them get out of bed, step out on the back porch (in winter), and cool the body down. Then when they return to bed they will be able to get back to sleep more easily. Another temperature related tip is to have a second place to sleep. If an adolescent awakens during the night on a regular basis and has trouble going back to sleep, have them move to another location. Move to that comfortable sofa or to a favorite recliner where they sometimes nap. First, it will initially be cooler than the bed they have been lying in. Second, the change in body position, the change in the resistance offered to the body, and the change in other tactile sensations will aid in getting back to slumber land.

The sense of smell can also play a part. Overpowering scents or acrid or foul odors certainly can keep us awake. Likewise, pleasant aromas can help us sleep. This is a good reason to have fresh sheets. For some children and adolescents it is incredibly important to address what scents they go to sleep with. I would recommend that we never underestimate the sense of smell. This sense, above all others, is processed directly by the limbic system, which is the emotional center of the brain. Smell can signify very quickly that we are in danger. Seeing smoke from a distance does not mean we are in danger, but if we smell smoke we are close enough that we had better react. Seeing a wild animal from a distance similarly does not necessarily evoke danger or threat in us. If we are close enough to smell the animal, however, we may be in trouble.

There is a story about an old physician who had a tremendous capability of diagnosing illnesses. He was incredibly accurate. Subsequent blood tests and other diagnostic tools typically proved him right. Why he was so good no one knew. Then one day he got a common cold. His sense of smell was not functional, and his skills at diagnosing illnesses suddenly went down the drain. He had been using his sense of smell as a diagnostic tool, but did not realize it. The point is, we cannot overlook scent or some sort of aromatherapy as a tool to help children sleep if they are having sleep problems.

There are some other things to consider in aiding sleep. Avoiding certain foods or substances before bed is crucial. High on the list of substances to avoid would include caffeine, nicotine, alcohol, spicy foods, or sugary foods. Some of these will keep us from sleep and some, like alcohol, might put us to sleep but cause us to wake up a few hours later and not be able to return to sleep. Additionally alcohol, as well as many street drugs and some prescription drugs, interferes with REM sleep. Consequently, even if sleep is attained it is not quality sleep.

It is also very helpful to get into a bedtime or nighttime routine. Don't alter the time for bed or the time for getting up significantly if that can be avoided. Get children and adolescents into a routine, for example, that ten o'clock is bedtime and six o'clock is wake time. The pattern, the routine will eventually begin to make them feel like they need to be in bed by ten o'clock because they are getting sleepy.

If their schedules permit, it is also valuable to use light and dark as the barometer for when they sleep. Our natural circadian rhythm is assisted and adjusted by light and darkness. If sleep is really a problem, make the effort to get the adolescent back into a natural circadian rhythm. It may take awhile to readjust if the cycle is way off, for example, a pattern of sleeping until noon or later, but the benefits gained by eventually getting the necessary sleep are well worth that effort.

In cases where the sleep cycle is way off, try adjusting it in small increments, like fifteen to twenty minutes a night. Don't try to make a huge adjustment because it simply won't work. Small adjustments will eventually get an adolescent back to a more natural routine.

Besides a regular time for bed, other bedtime routines can be helpful. The hour or so before bed get them into the habit of doing the same things. Bedtime preparations, teeth brushing, flossing, donning sleep attire, and a little reading is a great routine. By establishing a routine, that routine will start to signal the body to prepare for sleep.

While the routines for nighttime and for bed are critical, the other end of the sleep cycle is also critical. The wake-up time is a critical part of the routine. If we allow adolescents to sleep as late as they want, it becomes difficult to go to sleep at night when they need to. We mentioned going to bed earlier at night in fifteen or twenty-minute increments, but waking up earlier in fifteen or twenty-minute increments is just as important.

A final thought on routines concerns the snooze button on the alarm clock. Many adolescents have fallen in love with the snooze button. They are so tired and so constantly sleep deprived that they do not want to get out of bed when the alarm goes off. As a result some adolescents will set the alarm thirty minutes or so before they really need to get up just so they can lie there for another few minutes. In reality they are taking away the last thirty minutes or so of what could be good sleep. If they do that five days a week, that is another two and a half hours they really could have slept each week. It is better to not interrupt the last half hour of sleep. It is far better to set the alarm for when they really need to get up and allow for the extra thirty minutes of real sleep. Whatever we do, however, we cannot underestimate the power of routine.

A routine that should not be developed is the regular use of sleep medications. There is a difference between deep, restful sleep and being drugged. Many sleep medications, while they put us out, actually interfere with deep or slow wave sleep. As we have discussed earlier, slow wave sleep is incredibly important for a number of reasons, so merely putting ourselves into a state of unconsciousness is not all that productive.

While artificial sleep medications often interfere with slow wave sleep, melatonin is a natural sleep aid and is beneficial for some adults. Melatonin is naturally produced by our bodies to help us sleep. Because it is a natural substance many people have assumed that any side effects from its use must be benign. That is not necessarily the case for children and adolescents. While there is still much research that must be done, there are indications that melatonin use with children can delay the onset of puberty, impact seizure and epilepsy episodes, and exacerbate conditions such as asthma. Sleep deprivation is a serious concern, but the use of sleep medications is also a serious concern for children and adolescents. The point is the potential benefits must be carefully weighed against the potential harms before decisions are made in this regard.

When sleep won't come, don't continue to force the issue. That can become counter-productive. Instead, have the adolescent get up briefly, drink some warm milk, read a little, cool the body down, listen to a relaxation CD, and then try going back to bed.

For those who really are having difficulty sleeping it is also beneficial to keep a sleep journal. This should include writing down when they went to bed, when they think they awoke during the night and how often, when they got out of bed in the morning, and how much actual sleep they think they had. This would also include writing down whether they napped during the day, for how long they napped, and what time of the day they napped. Keeping such a journal can be enlightening as to what is really going on. This is also valuable information if we need to take a child to a sleep clinic.

If sleep just seems impossible to attain, or if a child seems to get enough sleep but still wakes up tired, it is time to seek medical advice. We should not allow our children to live long-term with sleep deprivation. While it is annoying, the ramifications of long-term sleep deprivation are far more severe than mere annoyance. It can have a significant impact on the physical health and mental health of our children.

A final strategy in helping us get more sleep concerns napping. Are naps good for us or bad for us? Some people love to nap and think it is wonderful, but some think it is a waste of time and, in fact, a negative in helping us sleep at night. Napping is such an interesting and complex subject that it deserves a chapter unto itself.

# Chapter 11

# The How, When, and Why of Napping

## *Creating the Perfect Nap*

*There was once a business manager who was concerned about his large staff. They worked hard and they always seemed busy, but they were having trouble meeting deadlines. They weren't getting the major projects completed on time. One morning at an impromptu staff meeting he brought in a large fish bowl. Into the fish bowl he first put some sand. After that he added some small pebbles. After that he tried to put in some larger rocks, but all the rocks wouldn't fit.*

*"Can anyone help me out here?" he asked.*

*"Sure," said several staff members in unison. "First take everything out of the fish bowl," they suggested and the manager did just that.*

*"Put the large rocks in first," they said, and the manager followed their directions.*

*"Next add the smaller pebbles," and so he did.*

*"Shake the fish bowl a little so the pebbles settle," came the directives and the manager eagerly complied.*

*"Now add in the sand."*

*As the manager added the sand he again shook the bowl slightly and the sand also settled between the rocks and pebbles and, to everyone's delight, it all fit in the bowl. He stared at the bowl for a moment and then produced a can of beer. He opened the beer and poured it into the bowl. The beer also went in nicely with no overflow. Then he turned to look at his staff.*

*"Just as we filled this fish bowl, we must fill our schedules with the big items first. If we fill our efforts with the small stuff there will never be room to get the big stuff in. If we make sure there is time and room for the big stuff, the rest can*

*be added and we will find a way to fit it in. There may even be room for an oc-*
*casional beer."*

*The same is true of napping. Some of us just don't have room in our schedules*
*for it. It we add it into our schedules first . . . if we make the room . . . it will fit*
*in nicely.*

What about napping? Some people think that napping during the day will keep us from sleeping at night, and therefore napping is a bad thing. Some physicians encourage people not to nap. Some of the most recent research does not agree with that. A designed nap at the right time of the day, for the right amount of time, will not interfere with our nocturnal sleep. Not only will it not interfere, but there is strong evidence that we are programmed for napping (Mednick 2006, 6). It is only in recent history that we have spurned the nap . . . and as a society we are showing the consequences of that. In this chapter we want to first discuss some elements of sleep and napping, and then apply this information to children and adolescents.

Sleep is cumulative. If we miss getting enough sleep one day we feel it the next. If we miss getting enough sleep for several days in a row we build up a sleep deficit. We have become a nation of sleep-deprived individuals because most of us do not get the sleep we need. Functioning with an ongoing sleep deficit results in slower reaction time, poor judgment, impaired information processing, impaired short term memory, impaired performance, loss of motivation, loss of vigilance, and loss of patience. We become people who are moody, aggressive, and burned out (Scott 2008). Sound like any adolescents you know?

One simple way to address this insidious sleep deprivation is through napping. In fact, we are one of very few species who do not nap routinely. One of the key reasons we do not nap is because we are so busy that we think our schedules have no room for napping. An interesting study was done in which individuals were cut off from the pressures of the outside world and lived in a sheltered environment for weeks at a time (Mednick 2006, 5–6). After a short period of adjustment they reverted to one long sleep period at night, and one short sleep period during the day. They were not directed to do this, but they would naturally put a nap into their day. This is natural because this is the way our bodies function.

Our sleep cycles, which are governed by two distinct impulses, drive not only how we sleep but also impact our waking states. We have a pressure that builds in us that requires slow wave sleep to sate that pressure, and we have the circadian cycle that dictates our REM sleep needs (Mednick , 2006, 46–49).

When we awaken in the morning we are at our most rested state and the need for, the pressure for, slow wave sleep is at its lowest. From the instant we awaken, however, that need for slow wave sleep begins to build. By bedtime we are ready for sleep because of this pressure. When this pressure is great enough we will sometimes go to sleep at the wheel of a car. Our bodies are telling us that we need sleep. . .specifically slow wave sleep.

In an earlier chapter it was discussed how slow wave sleep is critical to our health, to our very survival, because our immune systems will shut down without it. Hence, our bodies will put us into sleep even when we are desperately trying to fight it off, as when we are driving. This pressure is also the reason why we spend more time in slow wave sleep and less in REM sleep during the first few ninety-minute sleep cycles at night. As the need for slow wave sleep dissipates we get more REM sleep, which is what occurs in the later sleep cycles. The pressure to get slow wave sleep is very real and it is driven by our sleep behavior, i.e., by the time and amount of slow wave sleep we get.

In addition to this pressure, however, we also have the circadian rhythm. This is more like the effect of the moon on the tides. It is predictable by the time of day or night and is influenced by light and darkness. The circadian phase for REM sleep is at its peak generally about the time we arise in the morning and subsides throughout the day.

If we can picture this, the need for slow wave sleep is at its lowest ebb when we awaken and rises throughout the day. At the same time the need for REM sleep is at its peak when we arise and decreases throughout the day. Think of these two forces as lines on a continuum. One starts low and rises. The other starts high and falls. These two forces meet and cross each other during the day. In most of us that is somewhere around noon or one o'clock. Hence an hour nap around noon or so is the optimal time to get a relatively equal dose of both slow wave sleep and REM sleep. If we nap for an hour earlier than noon we will get more REM sleep, and if we nap much later than noon we will get more slow-wave sleep.

During nocturnal sleep our bodies will control the levels of sleep we attain. If we are healthy, not sleep deprived, and we get roughly eight hours of sleep, we will experience slow wave sleep and REM sleep in appropriate amounts. We cannot dictate when these come. . .they will come depending on our needs and sleep patterns. However, when we nap we certainly do influence what kind of sleep we will get. If we are sleep deprived we will get more slow-wave sleep because that pressure will take precedence. If we are not sleep deprived, however, the time we nap and the length of the nap will influence the type of sleep we get (Mednick 2006, 45).

An interesting aside is that some people state that they never dream. It is quite possible that some of those people are regularly sleep deprived. Hence they would spend more time in slow wave sleep rather than REM sleep, which would mean they don't dream as often because most dreams occur during REM sleep.

Another aspect of napping is how we feel after the nap. This is a critical factor. Some people don't like to nap because they feel sluggish afterwards. That is really an aspect of the length of nap and the stage of sleep we were in when we awoke rather than the nap itself. When we feel sluggish or feel what is termed "sleep inertia" upon awakening, it is because we have awakened out of a slow wave sleep cycle. Our brain waves are firing at a much slower rate during slow wave sleep (hence the name) and it takes a little time for them to adjust back to the waking state . . . hence the sluggishness. In level 2 sleep or REM sleep, the brain waves are much closer to the waking state and it is therefore easier and quicker for the brain to readjust to wakefulness.

The quick solution to that feeling of sluggishness is to either shorten or lengthen the nap time so as to awaken during level 2 or REM sleep. If, however, we are truly sleep deprived then the brain is under pressure to get slow wave sleep and will spend more time in slow wave sleep. Hence the likelihood of awakening in slow wave sleep and feeling sluggish increases for individuals who are chronically sleep deprived.

That being said, how can we design our nap time to achieve the greatest benefit? First, let's discuss the type of nap we are getting. Is it a planned nap, an emergency nap, or a habitual nap (National Sleep Foundation 2007)? The planned nap is the nap we take to avoid getting sleepy. If we know we are going to be up late that night, the planned nap beforehand can help get us through that period of time. This is a technique often practiced by college students and some adolescents who are planning to stay up very late Saturday night partying with friends, so they take a nap Saturday afternoon.

The emergency nap is just like it sounds. We take that nap because we are very tired and find it difficult to continue with whatever activity we are engaged in. This type of nap is often used by people who are driving through the night but become so tired they pull into a rest stop for a half hour emergency nap before continuing down the road.

The habitual nap is that nap that we take habitually each day, or many days, at around the same time each day. Young children take habitual naps regularly and far more often than adults, but there are numerous adults who have worked it into their busy schedules . . . particularly the after lunch nap. The schedules of most adolescents, at least during the school year, do not allow for napping unless it is a very late afternoon nap. A nap that occurs late in the afternoon and lasts for an hour or more will also begin to interfere with nocturnal sleep patterns. Many children, especially as they get older, will fight taking a nap. Wouldn't it be nice if a two-year-old said, "Gee, mom, I'm beat. I think I'll just take a little nap." Unfortunately, that doesn't happen. Adults who nap recognize the benefits, and we appreciate it.

The benefits of napping actually depend on the time of day we take a nap and the length of the nap taken. Mednick (2006, 97) gives a good description of the benefits of the different stages of sleep. The benefits of stage 2 sleep include a reduced level of sleepiness, an elevated mood, a boost in our alertness and attention, an increased ability to focus and concentrate, and better motor performance. These are not necessarily attributes we are consciously aware of after stage 2 sleep, but studies have proven that these benefits truly exist.

The main benefits of slow wave sleep (stages 3 and 4) include the fact that it acts to repair and restore our bodies, it enhances our immune system functioning, and it improves our declarative memory recall.

The benefits of REM sleep include an increased level of creativity, an increased ability to remember complex associative information, an improvement in the functioning of emotional memory, and better perceptual and sensory processing.

Understanding the benefits of the different stages allows us to understand napping. When we first go to sleep we go through a brief time in stage 1, and then spend roughly fifteen to seventeen minutes in stage 2. Consequently a twenty-minute nap will allow us to get mostly stage 2 sleep and reap some of the benefits mentioned above from that stage. That can pick us up, make us feel better and perform better, and keep us going.

If we get a longer nap, however, we can attain other benefits. If we get an hour nap, for example, and we get it around noon (assuming we are on a fairly typical wake/sleep schedule) we will get some stage 2 sleep and about an equal amount of slow wave sleep and REM sleep. If we nap much earlier than noon we will tend to get a little more REM sleep and a little less slow wave sleep. If we nap later in the afternoon we get less REM sleep and more slow wave sleep. Hence, we really can build designer naps based on what we are trying to accomplish. If we also build that nap into a routine or habitual nap, it becomes easier to go to sleep at that routine time.

So if we have decided to give napping a try, how do we improve our ability to nap? For adults, the first step is to plan the nap. The nap should not be stressful. We should not worry if we find it hard to get to sleep; just rest. We don't want to become more stressed that we are not sleeping when we have planned to sleep. This is not a sport, it is not a competition. If we build the habitual nap into our routine and continue to set aside that time, we will eventually begin to really nap during that allotted time.

The second step is to make a decision about when we are going to nap so it is a planned activity we can look forward to rather than feel guilty about taking. The decision as to when we take the nap should be partly determined by what we want to accomplish. That also includes planning how long we are going to nap. We should never (unless we are in a state of acute sleep deprivation) just take a nap and sleep until we wake up. That is a sure fire way to have a negative impact on nocturnal sleep. Planning the length of the nap can help us control whether it is just a twenty-minute power nap so we can function better, or whether it is a nap that gets us more slow wave or REM sleep.

By controlling the length of the nap we can also control whether we awaken during slow wave sleep, or awaken from stage 2 or REM sleep. As mentioned earlier, awakening during slow wave sleep is what gives us that unpleasant, sluggish, sleep inertia feeling.

The nap should also be in the right environment. That is sometimes hard to do, but finding a restful, quiet, dark spot can really enhance our ability to attain sleep. Closing the door to our room or office, turning off the lights, and spreading a yoga mat on the floor can do wonders.

While adults can plan a nap if we decide, even if it is merely taking twenty minutes of our lunch break, school age children and adolescents do not have that option in their schedules. For that option to exist, schools must create it. Additionally, because of time constraints, we can really only consider a twenty-minute power nap at school.

With that in mind, however, schools could create a safe, supervised room where students could take a twenty-minute nap as part of their lunch period. This should not be an enforced nap, but rather an option for students. It could and should be encouraged however. In some cases the length of the school day may need to be increased by fifteen to twenty minutes to accommodate this, but the benefits would soon become apparent. Students who took advantage of the nap option would be more alert, more focused, more attentive, less moody, and they would generally perform better on tasks and on tests during their afternoon classes. Their improved focus would also carry over to after-school practices for sports, drama, marching band, etc.

Setting up a lunchtime nap option for adolescents would require some work. Educators, school boards, and the public in general would have to be educated as to the need and the benefits of such a plan. That would be a challenge. Students might also be reluctant to use this option, at least initially. Consequently some education must be aimed at the student population.

Providing a quiet, supervised room where the lights are dimmed and there are cots available is also a necessity. The quietness of this room must be enforced by the adults on duty. Any student who is not quiet must leave. Nap start and ends times must be written on a dry-erase slate on each cot so the sleep attendant knows when to awaken each student. Basically, guidelines and rules must be set and adhered to, but the benefits would certainly be worth the effort.

Another issue that should be addressed in schools is that of the student who falls asleep in class. When this happens regularly it is a clear sign of sleep deprivation. Merely waking the student up does not solve the problem for the student or for the school. Even if he then remains awake he will not really be focused or attentive, so he is really not learning.

We need to address the sleeping student in two ways. First, send him to the nap room or nurse's office for a twenty-minute power nap. Second, a serious discussion needs to be held with the student and his parents. The parents need to understand what is happening and the parameters of that so as to address the nocturnal sleep patterns, and the student needs to understand what he is doing to his education by making the sleep related choices he is making. Some parents and some students won't respond to this, but some will.

For any student who does not respond, change his schedule. His first period in the morning should be in the nap-option room or the nurse's office. Let him sleep for an hour. That will sate his need for sleep and it will be harder for him to sleep the rest of the day. If he is awake for the rest of his classes he might also be able to focus and learn something. That is a better option than having him unfocussed all day long. We need to start addressing sleep as deprivation rather than as a reason for discipline.

Another consideration regarding napping is what we ingest. Just as caffeine can keep us up at night, it can also interfere with a nap. Coffee or other caffeine drinks can make napping impossible. If possible don't ingest caffeine for four hours before you nap. Have some right after the nap if you must, but don't ingest it beforehand. Also, foods such as turkey and cheese have higher levels of tryptophan which can be turned into melatonin in our bodies, so a light turkey and cheese sandwich can aid in our attempt to nap.

The question of flying across time zones is also important to address in this age when so many of us fly regularly. Some people advise us not to nap when we have flown across several time zones because it keeps our bodies from adjusting to the new time zone. That can happen if we take long naps. However, there are some steps we can take that will help (Mednick 2006, 113–14). The first is to allow ourselves to take a nap, but only a twenty minute nap. That allows us to get some needed stage 2 sleep, but is not long enough to get into the slow wave or REM sleep stages. If you are traveling with children or adolescents the same is true . . . allow them a twenty minute nap only. That will make them feel better and function better, but will not disrupt their ability to adjust to the new time zone.

Additionally, in preparation for such a trip, have them go to bed fifteen to twenty minutes earlier for a few nights if we are flying east, or go to bed fifteen minutes later if we are flying west. The wake up time should also be adjusted appropriately. This will act to give the circadian rhythm a boost in adjusting to the new time zone.

Napping can certainly be a key step in addressing sleep deprivation. For some groups it may be the best answer. For the elderly, who tend to get less nocturnal sleep for a variety of reasons, it is a way to get more of the sleep our bodies really need. Napping will not keep us from aging, but many of the supposed symptoms of aging including memory difficulties and bodily aches and pains can be somewhat mitigated if we get more REM and slow wave sleep. A daily nap of about an hour after lunch would accomplish that.

For adults, napping on the job (well maybe not on the job but at the work place) can also have multiple benefits. There are places around the world, and some places in the United States, where that is happening. Silicon Valley is one of them. We have discussed the benefits to the individual. The benefits to the company include the fact that napping reduces absenteeism, it increases productivity, it increases employee retention, and it saves money because it reduces wasted time and effort (Mednick 2006, 123). Although it has not been studied, companies which allow employees to nap will quite possibly find it ultimately decreases medical insurance claims because of the negative impact that sleep deprivation has on the immune system.

Since many people in our society are interested in the bottom line, the bottom line is this: we need to rethink our societal views on sleep and on napping. We need to make decisions based on research and logic rather than the American ideal that we can force our way through life by gutting it out. In the long run that ideal is neither healthy nor productive, and it is certainly not educationally nor economically sound. A sound nap is.

# Chapter 12

# Sleep and Our Society

## High School, Graduation Rates, Where Are We Headed?

*One day a traveler was walking down the road when he saw a monk working in a garden.*

*"Excuse me," said the traveler getting the monk's attention. "Is this the road to the village in the valley?"*

*"Yes it is," replied the monk.*

*"Could you tell me," continued the traveler, "what are the people like in the village?"*

*"Where are you coming from?" queried the monk.*

*"I am traveling from the village in the mountains," answered the traveler.*

*"And what were the people like there?" continued the monk.*

*"Oh, they were not a nice people. I am glad to be away from there. They were rude, and cold, and kept to themselves," replied the traveler.*

*"I am afraid you will find the people in the valley much the same," said the monk.*

*The traveler shook his head sadly and continued down the road.*

*Shortly there was another traveler coming down the same road. He too stopped to question the monk and was told this was the road to the village in the valley.*

*"And how are the people there?" asked the traveler.*

*"Where are you traveling from?" asked the monk.*

*"I am coming from the village in the mountains," replied the traveler.*

*"And how were the people there?"*

*"Oh, they were wonderful people. They were kind and generous, and I felt very much at home. I am sorry to have to leave there, but I will always have fond memories of my time there."*

*"You will find the people in the valley much the same," said the monk.*

*The traveler continued down the road and the monk turned to his disciple standing nearby and concluded the lesson thusly:*

*"The experiences we have in life greatly depend on what we ourselves bring to those experiences."*

We seem to have developed a culture where we don't sleep, where we believe that sleep is a waste of time, where we wear our sleep deprivation like a badge of honor. How little sleep can we get by on? We are also modeling this behavior for our children. We don't understand sleep and the result is not merely that we are not gaining the multiple benefits of sleep, but that we are actually doing harm to ourselves.

This seems especially true of industrialized countries. We are literally crippling our health. Cancer, diabetes, and other life threatening or life shortening illnesses that could be managed are literally killing us because our own immune systems are significantly neutralized because of sleep deprivation.

On January 17, 2008, there was a report on *Morning Edition* (National Public Radio) about sleep and how many people think it is a waste of time. One woman was quoted in the program whose daughter had a life threatening disease. They did not state what the disease was. What they reported was that the mother had asked the daughter if there was anything she could change, what would it be? The daughter's response was not what we might have expected, that she would be rid of the disease, but rather that she could abolish her need to sleep so she could get more done. We have to make the assumption that this young girl is getting as little sleep as she can get by on, and we then have to wonder if it was not the sleep deprivation that played a major role in either her getting sick or at least advancing the stage of her disease.

Granted, we really know nothing about this particular case. From what we do know about the importance of sleep for proper immune system functioning, however, there are cases like this that do not need to happen. Can we stop all disease by getting enough sleep? Of course not! We do know, however, that we can prevent a great deal of lung cancer by getting people to quit smoking, and in that same vein we could prevent or at least slow the progression of a great many diseases by getting people the sleep their bodies need.

Beyond the realm of illness and disease, our culture of cumulative sleep deprivation endangers the lives of others when we get behind the wheel of a car. This happens, and it happens a lot. It isn't merely that people will fall asleep behind the wheel, although that factor is enough for us to sit up and take notice. It is also that we make poor decisions, poor judgments, when we are tired. We think we can beat that other car and we risk lurching out in front of them as they are speeding down the road. A more rested brain would not attempt that same maneuver.

When we are sleep deprived we think we are functioning well, we report that we are functioning well, but the reality is that we are not functioning nearly as well as we function when we are rested. This disconnect in our thinking results in riskier decision making in all regards, and that includes behind the wheel of a vehicle. Statistics show that by far the highest percentage of fatalities from automobile accidents occur in the age group between sixteen and twenty-four. Statistics are also clear that the greatest cause of death for the fifteen to twenty-four age group is from accidents, and most of these accidents are automobile accidents.

Additionally, most adolescent accidents occur between the hours of two o'clock to five o'clock in the afternoon (after school) or after midnight. These are the times adolescents will be drowsy, and hence less focused and more apt to make poor decisions.

Beyond that, our own productivity and alertness are impacted by our lack of sleep. We do not respond as well or learn as well or as quickly when we suffer even minor amounts of sleep deprivation. We think we do, but the reality is that we don't.

Additionally, our attitude and behavior deteriorate when we are sleep deprived. Have you ever noticed that your own attitude is different when you are tired? That you are quick to snap at others, that you are simply more negative, that things get under your skin more rapidly when you are tired? How many child abuse incidents are directly the result of a parent who is tired from ongoing sleep deprivation and over-reacts to a situation?

If you are a parent of teenage children, have you noticed that they can become quite negative at times? They cop an attitude, so to speak. We also know that the majority of our teens are sleep deprived. How much of this negative, surly attitude is because of adolescence in general and how much is really related to sleep deprivation?

The point I have tried to make in this book is that sleep impacts us in many ways; that we need to get enough sleep for our physical, mental, emotional, and social well-being. Sleep is not a luxury that we can squander at a whim. Sleep is a necessity. The right amount and the proper quality of sleep are a necessity. Our productivity will not decrease if we are rested. We are not losing precious time that could be spent accomplishing something of vast importance. We will, in fact, be more efficient if we are well rested, and that means tasks can be accomplished more quickly with fewer errors.

Despite this growing base of knowledge, it is difficult to change old habits. Getting adults to change their sleep habits, while a worthy goal, will be a slow process at best. This is why we need to start early. We need to educate our children and adolescents about sleep and the importance of sleep. We need to provide the opportunity to take advantage of that knowledge, and we need to provide the structure to do so.

Besides the impact that sleep and the lack of sleep can have on children and adolescents individually, it also impacts us as a society. Quite literally our children are our future. There are some interesting studies that have been conducted regarding student achievement related to the time school begins.

The Center for Applied Research and Educational Improvement (Wahlstrom 2002) has led the way in some of this research. They studied two school corporations near Minneapolis, Minnesota, who changed their start times for high school students to about an hour later in the day. This study included over seven thousand students. Basically they found a reduction in drop-out rates, less depression, improved attendance, and somewhat higher grades. The attendance rates for students who were continuously enrolled in the same high school did not statistically change, but the attendance rates for the students who were not continuously enrolled in the same school improved significantly.

The majority of school administrators also reported calmer moods in the hallways and lunchrooms, less tardiness, and fewer disciplinary referrals. Parents reported fewer confrontations with their teens in the morning and basically improved family relationships.

Why would a later start time have beneficial effects on the education of adolescents? Research is showing that adolescents have a natural sleep pattern that results in a later-to-bed, later-to-rise cycle (Wahlstrom 2002). This is a result of the maturation of the endocrine system and the release of melatonin, and it is different for adolescents. Studies from multiple other countries revealed that the sleep-wake cycle for students in those countries was nearly identical to the cycles seen in students in the United States (Wahlstrom 2002, 19). In other words, the shift in the sleep cycles that we see in our adolescents is occurring in their neurological systems, not because of cultural influences.

The sleep patterns of adolescents are a phenomenon of human development, not because of laziness or because of culture. However, since our culture refuses to acknowledge that and continues to require teens to rise and go to school earlier than they are programmed to, we foster a system of sleep deprivation. Sleep deprivation leads to poor attendance, more drop-outs, poor graduation rates, higher rates of depression for adolescents, higher stress levels for adolescents, decreased ability to relate to adults including parents, and poor decision making which includes, by the way, decisions about alcohol and drugs. Educationally we are certainly paying the price for the sleep deprivation that we are fostering. Our teens are also paying the price.

We give lip service to improving graduation rates, but when it comes right down to doing something to actually help accomplish that, we often just flatly refuse to budge. Why does education exist in the first place? What are the most important factors? Do they include the education and well-being of our students, or are the most important factors the transportation schedules, the athletic schedules, or the preferences of some teachers to get home an hour earlier? What really drives our decisions?

Let's not put everything off on society and the school. There are things we can do with our own adolescents that are critical (National Public Radio 2007). The very first involves setting a strict turn off time for television, computers, phones, etc. One of the things that keeps adolescents awake is that they stay in touch, they stay connected with others in all manner of ways. The culture we live in includes television programming that never goes off the air, an Internet that is available twenty-four hours a day, seven days a week, and most teens that have their own cell phones for calling or text messaging each other at any time. This means that teens find it easy to stay up later and later. Having strict times when these means of connection must be off is critical to ensure sleep.

Some other strategies to help our teens would include scheduling early dinners. Many teens will skip the evening meal only to eat something very late at night. That can disrupt their ability to get to sleep. Hence, making sure they do eat at a regular and earlier mealtime is helpful in avoiding the late snack.

Another strategy is to help our teenagers develop a more natural and regular sleep–wake pattern. Part of that strategy might be to not allow them to sleep more than two hours later on weekends that they do during the week. This is difficult because they really are exhausted, but if they are allowed to sleep more than two extra hours on weekends, then Monday mornings become a real issue. A regular routine is critical for sleep, and hence for their health. The reasons for this should be explained to them, not merely imposed on them.

Along with establishing this wake up schedule, teens should be exposed to bright light when they get up. In the best of all possible situations teenagers should have rooms that face the east and have big windows with drapes. In the morning throw open the drapes to expose them to bright sunlight. If that is not possible, find a way to ensure they are exposed to bright light, even if it is artificial light, when they arise in the morning.

Other tips might include limiting caffeinated drinks, encouraging more exercise if they are not getting much, removing clutter from their rooms, allowing them to listen only to soft and soothing music at night, and making sure that all the preparations for the next day are done at night. That means homework is not only finished but in the backpack on the table ready to go for morning. It might mean that showers are taken the night before and that clothing for tomorrow is selected the night before and laid out ready to put on.

All the things that might be done to aid your teenager getting more and better sleep should be discussed with them beforehand. They need to understand the reasons why sleep is important, and they need to understand that the things you are doing are an attempt to ensure that they get the sleep they need. They may still resist the efforts to achieve this end, but knowing that there is a legitimate reason behind your actions will typically make it somewhat easier.

It is time we begin to recognize the real importance of sleep and the impact that being rested or being sleep deprived has on us as individuals and on us as a society. It affects our health, and it affects our health costs. It affects our attitude and outlook, and it affects how we get along with each other as a society. It affects whether a particular student drops out of school, and it affects our graduation rates. It affects our ability to learn, and it affects the number of engineers we can produce. It affects us now, and it certainly affects our future.

H. Jackson Brown, Jr., said "Opportunity dances with those who are already on the dance floor." We can truly impact the opportunities our children have, we can get them on the dance floor, by ensuring that they get the sleep they really need rather than just enough to get by on. The eventual price for sleep deprivation is high, while the opportunities that come from the proper quantity and quality of sleep are vast.

# References

Amen, D. G. (1998). *Change Your Brain Change Your Life: The Breakthrough Program for Conquering Anxiety, Depression, Obsessiveness, Anger, and Impulsiveness*. New York: Three Rivers Press.

Amen, D. G. (2002). *Mind Coach: How to Teach Kids and Teenagers to Think Positive and Feel Good*. Newport Beach, CA: Mindworks Press.

Cheng, M. (2007). "Graveyard Shift Soon to Be Listed as 'Probable' Cancer Cause." *Herald Times*, Associated Press Article, November 30, Nation & World section.

Coturnix (2005). "A Blog Around The Clock: (Non) Adaptive Function of Sleep." http://scienceblogs.com/clock/2006/10/non_adaptive_function_of_sleep.php.

Dweck, C. S. (2006). *Mindset: The New Psychology of Success*. New York: Random House, Inc.

Eichenbaum, H. B. (2004) "Brain Systems and Memory." Learning and the Brain Conference. Boston: Public Information Service.

Gilbert, D. T. (2002, November) "Why the Secret of Happiness Is a Secret to Adults and Children." Learning and the Brain Conference. Boston: Public Information Service.

Goldberg, E. (2001). *The Executive Brain: Frontal Lobes and the Civilized Mind*. New York: Oxford University Press, Inc.

Goleman, D. (1995). *Emotional Intelligence: Why It Can Matter More Than IQ*. New York: Bantam Books.

Greenfield, S. A. (1997). *The Human Brain: A Guided Tour*. New York: Basic Books.

Griffin, J. & Tyrrell, I. (2006). *Dreaming Reality: How Dreaming Keeps Us Sane, or Can Drive Us Mad*. Chalvington, East Sussex, United Kingdom: Human Givens Publishing, Ltd.

Hawkins, J. (2004). *On Intelligence: How a New Understanding of the Brain Will Lead To the Creation of Truly Intelligent Machines.* New York: Owl Books, Henry Holt and Company, LLC.

Johnson, S. (1998). *Who Moved My Cheese: An A-Mazing Way to Deal with Change in Your Work and in Your Life.* New York: G. P. Putnam's Sons.

Linden, D. J. (2007). *The Accidental Mind.* Cambridge, MA: The Belknap Press of Harvard University Press.

Lovre, C. (2004) "Workshop on Crisis Intervention, Trauma, and Stress." Crisis Management Institute. Bloomington, IN: National Education Service.

Lupine, S. J. (2004) "The impact of socioeconomic status on children's stress hormone levels, emotional processing, and memory performance." Learning and the Brain Conference. Boston: Public Information Resources.

Marshall, J. (2007). "To Sleep Perchance to Dream." *Zoogoer 36* (6). http://nationalzoo.si.edu/Publications/ZooGoer/2007/6/To_Sleep_Perchance_to_Dream.cfm.

Martin, P. (2002). *Counting Sheep: The Science and Pleasures of Sleep and Dreams.* New York: Thomas Duane Books, St. Martin's Griffin.

Mednick, S. C. (2006). *Take a Nap! Change Your Life.* New York: Workman Publishing.

National Public Radio (2007). "Helping Teens Make Peace with Sleep," *Morning Edition,* June 18, 2007. http://www.npr.org/templates/story.php?storyId=6894556.

National Public Radio (2008). "In Today's World, the Well-Rested Lose Respect," *Morning Edition,* January 17, 2008. http://www.npr.org/templates/story/story.php?storyId+18155047&sc=emaf

National Sleep Foundation (2007). "The Short Story on Napping." http://www.sleepfoundation.org/site/c.huIXKjMOIxF/b.2419153/k.8430/The_Short_Story_.

Parker, S. & Anderson, M. (2006). *212°: The Extra Degree.* Aurora, IL: Simple Truths.

Plaford, G. R. (2006). *Bullying and the Brain: Using Cognitive and Emotional Intelligence to Help Kids Cope.* Lanham, MD: Rowman & Littlefield Education.

Restak, R. (2003) *The New Brain: How the Modern Age Is Rewiring Your Mind.* Emmaus, PA: Rodale, Inc.

Scott, E. (2008). "Sleep Benefits: Power Napping for Increased Productivity, Stress Relief & Health." http://stress.about.com/od/lowstresslifestyle/a/powernap.htm.

Scripps Howard News Service (2008). "Weight Gain, Diabetes Linked to Lack of Sleep." *Herald Times.* Scripps Howard News Service, January 3, Nation & World section.

Siegel, J. M. (2005). "Clues to the Function of Mammalian Sleep." *Nature Publishing Group, 427* (27), 1272–78.

Siegel, J. M. (2001). "Hypothesis. Science," *294* (5544), 1058–63. http://www.npi.ucla.edu/sleepresearch/science/1058full.html.

Sjogren, B. & Robison, G.(2005). *Cat and Dog Theology: Rethinking Our Relationship with Our Master.* Colorado Springs, CO: Authentic Publishing.

Stickgold, R. (2005). "Sleep-dependent Memory Consolidation." *Nature Publishing Group, 437* (27), 1272–78.

Vertes, R. P. & Eastman, K. E. (2000). "The Case Against Memory Consolidation in REM Sleep," *Behavior Brain Science, 23* (867).

Wahlstrom, K. (2002). "Changing Times: Findings From the First Longitudinal Study of Later High School Start Times." *NASSP Bulletin 86* (633) December, 2002.

Wikipedia (2001). "Fibromyalgia." *The Free Encyclopedia.* http://en.wikipedia.ogr/wiki/Fibromyalgia.

———. "Growth Hormone." *The Free Encyclopedia.* http://en.wikipedia.ogr/wiki/Growth_Hormone.

———. "Hypothalamus." *The Free Encyclopedia.* http://en.wikipedia.ogr/wiki/Hypothalamus.

———. "Lymphatic System." *The Free Encyclopedia.* http://en.wikipedia.ogr/wiki/Lymphatic_system.

———. "Parasympathetic System." *The Free Encyclopedia.* http://en.wikipedia.ogr/wiki/Parasympathetic nervous system.

Winstead, E. R. (2001). "Two Studies on Schizophrenia and Motion Perception." *Genome News Network.* http://www.genomenewsnetwork.org/articles/12_01/Schizophrenia_motion.shtml.

# Index

# About the Author

**Gary Plaford** served as director of the Social Service Department for the Monroe County Community School Corporation from 1986 until his retirement in 2007. He supervised a staff of fifteen MSW social workers. He continues to teach social work classes through Indiana University in Bloomington on understanding and dealing with youth and adolescents and on dealing with organizations. He has written a book *Bullying and the Brain* that was released in 2006 through Rowman & Littlefield Publishers. In May 2007 he spoke at the Learning and the Brain Conference in Boston, Massachusetts, on the topic of bullying and the brain. In July 2007 he spoke on the topic of Poverty and the Brain at the Oxford Round Table at the University of Oxford, Oxford, England. He has made multiple presentations at state conferences such as at the Indiana School Safety Specialist Academy, the NASW state conference, and the Indiana Counseling Association state conference, and has spoken to combinations of administrators, faculty, and staff at numerous schools around Indiana.